BROMOCRIPTINE

A Clinical and Pharmacological Review

Bromocriptine

A Clinical and Pharmacological Review

Michael O. Thorner, M.B., M.R.C.P.

Department of Internal Medicine
University of Virginia
School of Medicine
Charlottesville, Virginia

E. Flückiger, Dr. sc. nat.

Preclinical Research
Pharmaceutical Division
Sandoz Ltd.
Basel, Switzerland

Donald B. Calne, D.M., F.R.C.P.

National Institute of Neurological and Communicative Disorders and Stroke
National Institutes of Health
Bethesda, Maryland

Raven Press ■ New York

Raven Press, 1140 Avenue of the Americas, New York, New York 10036

Made in the United States of America

International Standard Book Number 0–89004–419–8
Library of Congress Catalog Card Number 79–64424

Great care has been taken to maintain the accuracy of the information contained in the volume. However, Raven Press cannot be held responsible for errors or for any consequences arising from the use of the information contained herein.

Dr. Calne has coauthored this volume in his private capacity and not as part of his duties as a U.S. Government appointee.

Preface

Bromocriptine is the first in a new class of drugs, the dopamine agonists. It was developed as a specific inhibitor of prolactin release from the anterior pituitary, and it was only after its introduction into clinical research that it was recognized to act through dopamine mechanisms. Several more years elapsed before dopamine came to be considered the most important physiological hypothalamic prolactin release inhibiting factor.

Research in pharmacology, neurophysiology, endocrinology, and clinical therapeutics has advanced so rapidly that many physiologists and clinicians not working directly in these fields may feel left behind. It is the aim of this volume to review some aspects of the pertinent physiology of dopamine mechanisms, both within and outside the central nervous system; the pharmacology of bromocriptine; and for those unfamiliar with disorders of prolactin secretion, the pathophysiology and clinical features of hyperprolactinemia. The first 9 years of clinical research with bromocriptine, both in endocrinology and neurology, are reviewed. Some future applications of bromocriptine and other dopamine agonists are discussed.

This volume is written primarily for the clinician—whether endocrinologist, neurologist, obstetrician and gynecologist, psychiatrist, or general physician—and will serve as a current state of the art for researchers in the field. It will not only aid in the understanding of the many different indications for the use of bromocriptine, but will hopefully open new frontiers in physiology and pathophysiology.

Contents

1

The Interrelationship of the Nervous and Endocrine Systems and the Role of Dopamine Agonist Drugs

I. INTRODUCTION

Bromocriptine was developed as an orally effective drug specifically to inhibit prolactin release (9). At the time it was developed, its mode of action was unknown; and although it is now clear that it acts through dopamine mechanisms, the molecular steps that occur within the cell following binding of the drug to the receptor on the cell surface are still unknown. Until 1970 the very existence of prolactin in man was questioned, since growth hormone was considered to be the human lactogenic hormone. At the same time that bromocriptine was being developed, prolactin was identified as a separate and distinct anterior pituitary hormone in man. Shortly thereafter, Friesen and colleagues isolated pure human prolactin, which made possible the development of specific and sensitive radioimmunoassays for the measurement of human prolactin (15). These assays allowed the study of the physiology of prolactin secretion, and were also instrumental in identifying hyperprolactinemia as the most common hypothalamic pituitary disorder in clinical practice (10,11,29). Thus, an endocrine disorder was uncovered at the time that a drug became available to treat the condition. After the drug had been in use in clinical research for 2 or 3 years, it was shown to act by stimulating dopamine receptors (2,12), and in another 2 or 3 years the hypothalamic prolactin inhibiting hormone was identified as the catecholamine dopamine (24).

In this volume we have attempted to bring together both laboratory and clinical results from experience with this exciting compound—bromocriptine. It is clearly the first of a new class of compounds that act by stimulating dopamine receptors. In retrospect, the story can be united under the concept of stimulation of dopamine receptors by bromocriptine. The various indications for this compound evolved in two different ways: first, it was developed as a specific inhibitor of prolactin secretion, and second, the later discovery of bromocriptine's ability to stimulate dopamine receptors led logically to its application in the treatment of parkinsonism and acromegaly.

Before proceeding further, it may be useful to review current ideas concerning the relationship between the nervous and endocrine systems, since bromocriptine has found useful application in both clinical endocrinology and in neurology.

II. RELATIONSHIP BETWEEN THE NERVOUS AND ENDOCRINE SYSTEMS

Claude Bernard stressed the importance of maintaining homeostasis—to maintain the *milieu interieur.* For a complex organism with specialized tissues to achieve this, a highly sophisticated system of control is necessary to integrate the multicellular, multitissue, and multiorgan systems so that the organism can sustain itself in the face of the changing environment. At its simplest this involves the reaction of a unicellular organism, e.g., chemotaxis of an ameba. As vertebrates evolved, specialized neural tissues have developed to integrate the functions of the organism. Classically, it was considered that the neural system was one in which responses were rapid, while the endocrine system was a slower and more gradual control system; however, even this distinction is no longer clear-cut.

Pearse and Takor (22) have proposed that the nervous system be subdivided into three branches:

1. Somatic (motor and sensory);
2. Autonomic (sympathetic and parasympathetic); and
3. Endocrine (central neuroendocrine and peripheral).

All three branches are derived from neuroectoderm. This concept is generally accepted regarding the first two, but the endocrine division is controversial. However, the observations on which these workers based their classification were drawn from morphological studies that demonstrated that certain peptide-secreting cells had APUD characteristics—*A*mine content, Amine *P*recursor *U*ptake, and enzymes to *D*ecarboxylate. Although certain peptide-secreting cells have lost some of the APUD characteristics, embryological studies suggest that all peptide-secreting cells are derived from neuroectoderm (22).

Thus, the nervous system, in its broadest sense, incorporates not only classic neurotransmission but also neurosecretion of both neurotransmitters and hormones. The similarity in the process of neurotransmitter release at a synapse and hormone secretion has been stressed by Douglas in his elegant studies on secretion coupling (7). The concept of neurotransmission being electrical in nature is also true for at least some endocrine cells in which action potentials are associated with hormone secretion (5,6,8,19–21,26). Thus depolarization of endocrine cells leads to hormone release, which is analogous to the process of neurotransmitter release from neurons.

The distinction between a neurotransmitter and a hormone does not depend on structure, but on the manner of secretion. In practice, three patterns of neurosecretion may be described to distinguish three types of control (Fig. 1):

1. Classic neurotransmitters are released from neurons into synaptic clefts to produce excitatory or inhibitory postsynaptic potentials at the adjacent neuron, thus affecting its function. The effects of peripheral nerves on their target organs, e.g., blood vessels, muscle, or secretory tissue, are mediated by similar processes.
2. Hormones are released from endocrine cells (which may retain neuronal characteristics, e.g., hypothalamic dopaminergic or peptidergic neurons) into the bloodstream to affect cells at a distant site with specific receptors. They can therefore have widespread and specific effects, e.g., epinephrine in the "flight and fight" stress response, and corticotropin on the adrenal cortex.
3. Paracrine hormones are released from endocrine cells into the extracellular fluid. They diffuse locally—outside the circulatory system—to affect function of adjacent cells, e.g., somatostatin in the endocrine pancreas and in the wall of the gut. These points can be illustrated by considering the catecholamines epinephrine

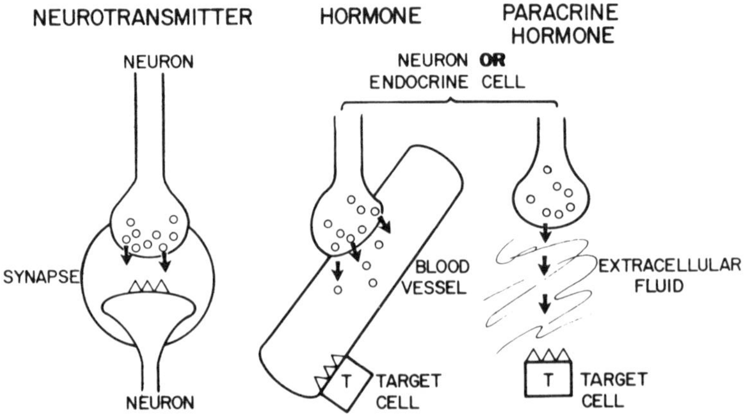

FIG. 1. Diagrammatic representation of characteristics and similarities of neurotransmitters, hormones, and paracrine hormones.

and norepinephrine, which, within the central nervous system, act as classic neurotransmitters but when released from the adrenal medulla act as hormones. In the periphery dopamine has been considered a precursor of epinephrine and norepinephrine and also a classic neurotransmitter in the brain; more recently it has been considered to be a hormone as well—a prolactin-inhibiting hormone. It is secreted by the hypothalamic tuberoinfundibular dopamine neurons and is released from their nerve endings, at the median eminence, into the portal capillaries, through which it is transported to the pituitary. There it inhibits prolactin release from the lactotroph cells (18,29). Somatostatin, a tetradecapeptide, was isolated from the hypothalamus as the regulatory hormone for inhibiting growth hormone release. However, it very rapidly became apparent that it was capable of inhibiting the release of many hormones. It is widely distributed in the central nervous system and in the endocrine pancreas and gut (17,23). In the central nervous system it presumably acts as a classic neurotransmitter, and in the hypothalamus as a hormone to be released into the portal capillaries and transported to the pituitary to inhibit growth hormone release. In the pancreas and gut it acts as a paracrine hormone; it is released and affects cells locally, but does not have widespread effects because of its limited diffusion.

Thus, the overlap of the somatic, autonomic, and endocrine divisions of the nervous system are clear. The highly sophisticated control depends on selective release of neurotransmitters, including hormones; specificity both of the neurotransmitter and its target receptors; and finally, the selective distribution of the neurotransmitter, e.g., at the synapse, into portal capillaries, into the general circulation, or into the extracellular fluid.

III. DOPAMINE MECHANISMS

It is beyond the scope of this volume to review the role of dopamine in the body, but a few comments may be useful in putting into context the widespread effects of bromocriptine.

Dopamine is secreted by a series of neurons. Specific dopamine pathways have been mapped in the rat brain by Fuxe and colleagues, who used histochemical techniques (13). These workers have described three major pathways:

1. Nigro-neostriatal dopamine neurons;
2. Mesolimbic dopamine neurons; and
3. Tuberoinfundibular dopamine neurons in the hypothalamus.

These three major pathways subserve motor, mental (and behavioral), and endocrine functions, respectively. Outside the central nervous system, dopamine pathways are more difficult to locate. However, considerable levels of dopamine are found in a wide variety of tissues, and it seems likely that dopamine has a significant role not only in the central nervous system, but also in the autonomic nervous system, the spinal cord, the gut, and the exocrine pancreas. It also acts as a hormone in controlling vascular tone. Dopamine's role in the control of hypothalamic-pituitary function is discussed in Chapters 2, 3, and 4 of this volume. It is likely that dopamine is important not only in controlling prolactin secretion but also in controlling the release of several hypothalamic regulatory hormones. The identification of specific dopamine receptors in a variety of tissues outside the central nervous system is one of the most compelling arguments to support the concept that dopamine has an important physiological role in the periphery. The effects of catecholamines have in the past been considered to be mediated through α and β adrenoreceptors. However, dopamine receptors are distinct from these and have been identified in the renal, mesenteric, coronary, and cerebral vascular trees, in kidney and exocrine pancreas, and in the brain and pituitary (14,28).

A final level of dopaminergic discrimination is at the receptor site. Accumulating evidence indicates that multiple types of dopamine receptors exist. The dopamine ergot derivatives have proved to be useful tools for the analysis of separate receptor mechanisms, since they are potent agonists for certain phenomena mediated by dopamine (e.g., prolactin suppression), whereas they are either inactive or antagonistic in other pharmacological responses to dopamine (e.g., stimulation of cyclic AMP formation in homogenates of the caudate nucleus). While various criteria can be employed to formulate a classification of dopamine receptors, recent proposals (16) have suggested a major subdivision based on whether or not the receptors are linked to an adenylate cyclase. This approach yields two categories of receptors, analogous to the α and β norepinephrine receptors and the H-1 and H-2 histamine receptors. Those dopamine receptors that are associated with an adenylate cyclase have been designated as D-1 type, and those that are independent of a cyclase have been termed D-2 type. Other features of this classification are summarized in Table 1.

It is evident that cyclic AMP can be regarded as a "second messenger" for D-1 receptors, just as it is for β adrenergic receptors and H-2 histamine receptors. This analysis of dopaminergic receptor organization is still at an early stage of development.

TABLE 1. *Criteria for the classification of dopamine receptors*

Name	D-1	D-2
Cyclase linkage	Yes	No
Location of prototype receptor	Bovine parathyroid	Mammotroph of anterior pituitary
Dopamine	Agonist (μmolar potency)	Agonist (nmolar potency)
Apomorphine	Partial agonist or antagonist	Agonist (nmolar potency)
Dopaminergic ergots	Potent antagonist (nmolar potency) Weak agonist (μmolar potency)	Agonist (nmolar potency)
Selective antagonist	None known as yet	Metoclopramide sulpiride
Radiolabeled ligand	*cis*-Flupenthixol[a]	Dihydroergocryptine

[a] Radiolabeled *cis*-flupenthixol can be used as a ligand specific for the dopamine receptor linked to adenylyl cyclase in the rat striatum. Its affinity for the dopamine receptor in the anterior pituitary has not been measured.

Reproduced from Kebabian and Calne; ref. 16, with permission.

Further evidence must be acquired before it is possible to confirm or refute the value of subdividing dopamine receptors on the basis of their relationship with cyclic nucleotides.

The commonest disorder of dopamine mechanisms in man is seen in parkinsonism. In Parkinson's disease, anatomical lesions in the basal ganglia are found; these are associated with destruction of dopamine neurons. It is likely that there are other disorders of dopamine in man. Recently, Van Loon has described one such abnormality in patients with prolactin-secreting pituitary tumors (30). He has shown that in normal men a single 2.5 mg dose of bromocriptine will lead to suppression of catecholamines to $33 \pm 5\%$ of control for plasma dopamine, $33 \pm 5\%$ for plasma epinephrine, and $37 \pm 3\%$ for norepinephrine, 2 hr following the dose. When he repeated the study in 5 patients with hyperprolactinemia and in 2 patients 1 year after removal of a prolactin-secreting tumor, he found that their basal levels of catecholamines were normal, and that bromocriptine did not lead to the decline in catecholamine levels. On the basis of these observations he has postulated that in patients who harbor, or have harbored, a prolactin-secreting tumor, the basic defect involves catecholamines, such that negative feedback is absent. Thus, the abnormality leading to hyperprolactinemia is in the hypothalamic catecholamine neurons, which leads to excessive prolactin secretion, hyperplasia, and/or adenoma formation of the lactotrophs (30). This proposal is exciting and will certainly be studied further.

IV. HISTORICAL REVIEW OF DRUGS USED IN INCREASING DOPAMINERGIC TONE

Attempts to increase dopaminergic transmission began in 1961, following the identification of dopamine as a transmitter that became depleted in the brain of parkinsonian patients. Since dopamine does not readily cross the blood-brain barrier, its immediate precursor, levodopa, was administered. The dramatic therapeutic action of high doses of levodopa in parkinsonism was followed by a critical evaluation of its adverse effects, and so new approaches to treatment were sought. Substances that mimicked dopamine at synaptic receptors, termed direct agonists, were investigated as adjuvants or alternatives to levodopa.

The first artificial dopamine agonist to be studied was apomorphine. Prior to the recognition of its dopamine agonist properties, Schwab et al. (25) reported its beneficial actions. This observation was confirmed and extended by Cotzias et al. (3), who were aware of the dopamine agonist properties of apomorphine, but they found that this drug induced unacceptable nephrotoxicity. These workers attempted to identify a congener that would be better tolerated, and initially reported encouraging results with *N*-propyl-noraporphine (4). Although less toxic than apomorphine, *N*-propyl-noraporphine still impaired renal function, so its use was abandoned.

Another dopaminergic agonist that underwent clinical study was piribedil (1). A similar experience emerged: piribedil was therapeutically active in parkinsonism, but adverse reactions—primarily psychiatric side effects—precluded its widespread introduction (1).

V. DEVELOPMENT OF OTHER DOPAMINE AGONISTS

Although bromocriptine fulfills many of the requirements for an ideal dopamine agonist, it does have marked adverse reactions when taken in high doses for the treatment of acromegaly, and more particularly for parkinsonism, where the patients comprise an older and sicker group. Furthermore, the synthesis of bromocriptine is complex and expensive; therefore, the cost of the drug, particularly when given in large doses, becomes extremely high, and this limits its widespread use. For these reasons, other, newer synthetic ergots, without peptide side chains (ergolines), are being developed. It is hoped that these compounds will have: (a) a higher therapeutic index (particularly in parkinsonism); (b) an even longer duration of action, to permit a once-daily regimen; and (c) less expensive production, which would lower the cost to the patient.

One of the challenges in developing dopaminergic agonists for treatment of parkinsonism and pituitary disorders is designing drugs with specificity for either site of action. This could be achieved by confining the distribution of the drug to one or other side of the blood-brain barrier, or by identifying distinct receptors with different characteristics at each site. If the latter were true, then it should be possible to develop drugs that would be specific for each site. However, at present it appears that all drugs that are effective in treating parkinsonism are also very potent in inhibiting prolactin release. In Chapter 2 *(this volume),* the pharmacologic actions of bromocriptine are reviewed, but it is worth stressing that the effects of the extrapyramidal model systems parallel those at the pituitary—thus, perhaps at present, the simplest predictive test for clinical efficacy of dopamine agonists is their ability to suppress prolactin release.

Another major problem in developing new dopaminergic agents is the inadequacy of predictive tests for some of the salient adverse reactions these drugs can induce. This dilemma is seen most clearly in the context of antiparkinsonism therapy, where high doses are employed and the patients tend to be elderly and more vulnerable to adverse effects. The problem can be resolved into (a) difficulty in establishing a laboratory homologue of human adverse reaction, and (b) interspecies variation.

(a) Difficulty in establishing a laboratory analogue of adverse reactions and toxicity. This is exemplified by the failure to establish any behavioral or biochemical laboratory correlates for such important unwanted effects as psychiatric reactions (hallucinations and delusions) and the erythromelalgic syndrome (p. 150). There is even uncertainty over dyskinesia; it is not clear whether this reaction is best represented in animals by stereotypic behavior, increased locomotor activity, or induction of rotation following unilateral lesions of the nigro-striatal pathway.

(b) Interspecies variation. Conventional toxicological studies provide obvious paradigms for screening such toxic reactions as hepatocellular injury. However, there are notable examples of dopaminergic ergot derivatives causing such problems in man

despite their "safety" having been demonstrated in a battery of preliminary studies in animals. Thus, lergotrile (an ergoline) fails to display hepatotoxic properties in rodents, dogs, or nonhuman primates; in man, over 50% of parkinsonian patients have reportedly developed evidence of hepatic damage (27).

Because of the difficulty in establishing predictive tests for adverse reactions to dopaminergic ergots, extensive studies in man are necessary, with particularly cautious surveillance for adverse effects. As new compounds are screened clinically in this way, it should prove possible to amass sufficient documented experience to discern some correlation between the different pharmacological profiles of activity in animals and man. Currently, two new dopaminergic ergots—lisuride and pergolide—are being investigated in this way. Since neither of these compounds has peptide side chains, they would have the practical advantage over bromocriptine of being considerably less expensive. However, they will have to be shown to be at least as good as bromocriptine to be adopted for use in clinical practice. At present, bromocriptine is the yardstick with which these compounds are to be compared.

REFERENCES

1. Calne, D., Chase, T. N., and Barbeau, A., editors (1975): *Advances in Neurology, Vol. 9: Dopaminergic Mechanisms.* Raven Press, New York.
2. Corrodi, H., Fuxe, K., Hökfelt, T., Lidbrink, P., and Ungerstedt, U. (1973): Effect of ergot drugs on central catecholamine neurons: Evidence for a stimulation of dopamine neurons. *J. Pharm. Pharmacol.,* 25:409–412.
3. Cotzias, G. C., Papvasilious, P. S., Fehling, C., Kaufman, B., and Mena, I. (1970): Similarities between neurologic effects of L-Dopa and apomorphine. *N. Engl. J. Med.,* 1:31–33.
4. Cotzias, G. C., Papvasilious, P. S., Tolosa, E. S., Mendex, J. S., and Bell-Midura, M. (1976): Treatment of Parkinson's disease with apophines. Possible role of growth hormone. *N. Engl. J. Med.,* 11:567–572.
5. Dean, P. M., and Mathews, E. K. (1970): Glucose induced electrical activity in pancreatic islet cells. *J. Physiol.,* 210:255–264.
6. Dean, P. M., and Mathews, E. K. (1970): Electrical activity in pancreatic islet cells: Effects of ions. *J. Physiol.,* 210:265–275.
7. Douglas, W. W. (1974): Mechanisms of release of neurohypophyseal hormones: Stimulus-secretion coupling. In: *Handbook of Physiology, Vol. 14: The Pituitary Gland and its Neuroendocrine Control, Part 1,* edited by E.

Knobil and W. H. Sawyer, pp. 191–224. American Physiological Society, Washington, D.C.

8. Douglas, W. W., and Taraskevich, P. S. (1978): Action Potentials in gland cells of rat pituitary pars intermedia: Inhibition by dopamine, an inhibitor of MSH secretion, *J. Physiol.,* 285:171–184.
9. Flückiger, E., and Wagner, H. (1968): 2-Br-α-ergokryptin; Beeinflussung von Fertilität and Laktation bei der Ratte. *Experientia,* 24:1130–1131.
10. Franks, S., Murray, M. A. F., Jequier, A. M., Steele, S. J., Nabarro, J. D. N., and Jacobs, H. S. (1975): Incidence and significance of hyperprolactinemia in women with amenorrhoea. *Clin. Endocrinol. (Oxf.),* 4:587–607.
11. Franks, S., Nabarro, J. D. N., and Jacobs, H. S. (1977): Prevalence and presentation of hyperprolactinemia in patients with "functionless" pituitary tumors. *Lancet,* 1:778–780.
12. Fuxe, K., Corrodi, H., Hökfelt, T., Lidbrink, P., and Ungerstedt, U. (1974): Ergocornine and 2-Br-α-ergocryptine. Evidence for prolonged dopamine receptor stimulation. *Med. Biol.,* 52:121–132.
13. Fuxe, K., Hökfelt, T., and Ungerstedt, U. (1970): Morphological and functional aspects of central monoamine neurons. *Int. Rev. Neurobiol.,* 13:93–126.
14. Goldberg, L. I. (1975): Commentary: The dopamine vascular receptor. *Biochem. Pharmacol.,* 24:651–653.
15. Hwang, P., Guyda, H., and Friesen, H. (1971): A radioimmunoassay for human prolactin. *Proc. Natl. Acad. Sci. U.S.A.,* 68:1902–1906.
16. Kebabian, J. W., amd Calne, D. B. (1979): Multiple receptors for dopamine. *Nature,* 277:93–96.
17. Luft, R., Efendic, S., Hökfelt, T., Johansson, O., and Arimura, A. (1974): Immunohistochemical evidence for localisation of somatostatin-like immunoreactivity in a cell population of the pancreatic islets. *Med. Biol.,* 52:428–430.
18. MacLeod, R. M. (1976): Regulation of prolactin secretion. In: *Frontiers in Neuroendocrinology, Vol. 4,* edited by L. Martini and W. F. Ganong, pp. 169–194. Raven Press, New York.
19. Mathews, E. K., and Sakamoto, Y. (1975): Electrical characteristics of pancreatic islet cells. *J. Physiol.,* 246:421–437.
20. Meissner, H. P., and Schmelz, H. (1974): Membrane potential of beta-cells in pancreatic islets. *Pflügers Arch.,* 351:195–206.
21. Pace, C. S., and Price, S. (1974): Bioelectrical effects of hexoses on pancreatic islet cells. *Endocrinology,* 94:142–147.
22. Pearse, A. G. E., and Takor, T. (1976): Neuroendocrine embryology and the APUD concept. *Clin. Endocrinol.,* 5:229s–244s.
23. Polak, J. M., Pearse, A. G. E., Grinnelius, L., Bloom, S. R., and Arimura, A. (1975): Growth-hormone releasing inhibiting hormone (GH-RIH) in gastrointestinal and pancreatic D cells. *Lancet,* 1:1220–1222.
24. Schally, A. V., Dupont, A., Arimura, A., Takahara, J., Redding, T. W., Clemens, J., and Shaar, C. (1976): Purification of catecholamine-rich fraction with prolactin release-inhibiting factor (PIF) activity from porcine hypothalami. *Acta Endocrinol. (Kbh.),* 82:1–14.

25. Schwab, R. S., Amador, L. V., and Lettvin, J. Y. (1951): Apomorphine in Parkinson's disease. *Trans. Am. Neurol. Assoc.,* 76:251–263.
26. Taraskevich, P. S., and Douglas, W. W. (1977): Action potentials occur in cells of the normal anterior pituitary gland and are stimulated by the hypophysiotropic peptide thyrotropin-releasing hormone. *Proc. Natl. Acad. Sci. U.S.A.,* 74:4064–4067.
27. Teychenne, P. F., Jones, E. A., Ishak, K. G., and Calne, D. B. (1979): Hepatocellular injury with distinctive mitochondrial changes induced by lergotrile mesylate: A dopaminergic ergot derivative. *Gastroenterology,* 76:575–583.
28. Thorner, M. O. (1975): Dopamine is an important neurotransmitter in the autonomic nervous system. *Lancet,* 1:662–664.
29. Thorner, M. O. (1977): Prolactin: Clinical physiology and the significance and management of hyperprolactinemia. In: *Clinical Neuroendocrinology,* edited by L. Martini and G. M. Besser, pp. 319–361. Academic Press, New York.
30. Van Loon, G. R. (1978): A defect in catecholamine neurons in patients with prolactin secreting adenomas. *Lancet,* 2:868–871.

2

The Pharmacology of Bromocriptine

I. INTRODUCTION

Shelesnyak, studying the mechanism of ovum implantation in the rat (151), was the first to note that certain ergot alkaloids suppress prolactin secretion. Describing his observations in 1954 (150), he concluded that they could act either through the hypothalamus or directly on the pituitary. Later, Zeilmaker and Carlsen (176) elegantly showed that one of these alkaloids, ergocornine, acts at the pituitary level. The observations of Shelesnyak had expanded the known spectrum of activity of ergot alkaloids (9,22,137) in an unexpected way. The question arose whether or not this new property was clinically relevant and how it was related to the "classical" activities of ergot alkaloids. Therefore, a systematic pharmacological study of ergot alkaloids and ergot derivatives began in the early sixties, with the goal of finding a compound suitable for clinical use as an inhibitor of prolactin secretion. This work was handicapped by a lack of methods for measuring prolactin in blood. Hence, the inhibitory potency of test compounds on prolactin secretion was assessed with the aid of bioassay procedures, such as interruption of leukocyte dominance in vaginal smears of pseudopregnant rats or inhibition of ovum implantation in inseminated rats. These methods have the practical advantage of excluding short-acting drugs (42,43). Another method that became very important in the early phase of this work was the suppression of lactation, an indicator of prolactin secretion that could first be used in various mammalian species (40) and later, in the clinic (95,164). As a result of these pharmacological studies (38,46,49), 2-Br-α-ergokryptine mesylate (CB 154) [bromocriptine mesylate (U.S. Approved Name)]—the active principle in Parlodel® and Pravidel® (141)—was selected in 1967 for development as a therapeutic agent. Although many analogs have been tested, bromocriptine remains the best characterized and clinically most useful compound of its class (42,48). From 1969 onward, bromocriptine was offered to numerous investigators as a tool for their special research projects. In many cases the drug proved to be a valuable probe in elucidating various endocrine and neurologic problems, and in return, the results from such studies contributed in a very important way to the biological characterization of this drug.

II. ENDOCRINE ACTIONS

A. Inhibition of Prolactin Secretion

Bromocriptine inhibits prolactin secretion in females and males of all species of fish and mammals tested so far (39) under basal conditions or under conditions in which hormone output is stimulated by physiological, pharmacological or surgical means.

1. Sites of Action

Bromocriptine inhibits prolactin secretion when added to pituitaries *in vitro* or to pituitary cell cultures (84,119,123,158,168, 175). This is unambiguous evidence of a direct action on the prolactin cell. *In vivo* experience also suggests a direct action on the pituitary; since bromocriptine blocks TRH stimulation of prolactin secretion (139), it suppresses serum prolactin levels in the presence of an ectopic pituitary (46) and it normalizes elevated serum prolactin levels of rats pretreated with reserpine and α-methyl-p-tyrosine (41). It is not clear whether, in the intact rat, bromocriptine also acts at the hypothalamic level (71) to enhance inhibition of prolactin secretion. Changes in serum prolactin levels have a feedback action on transmitter turnover in the median eminence (37,51,122).

2. *Mechanism of Action*

Bromocriptine reduces prolactin secretion not by an immediate attenuation of hormone synthesis (172,173) but by reducing exocytotic events (70). This is accompanied in a first phase by an increase in pituitary prolactin (44,70,83,158,173). Prolonged treatment of mice with bromocriptine produced a reduction of pituitary prolactin content and concentration (171,172), indicating that suppression of hormone release over an extended period of time leads to changes in the metabolism of the prolactin cell. These aspects have attracted little attention to date. When treating male rats continuously with estrogens, concomitant bromocriptine treatment produced lower serum prolactin levels, diminished DNA synthesis, and reduced mitotic activity in the pituitary (32,90,91). This seems to signify that continued suppression of prolactin release may lead to attenuation of cell metabolism and mitotic processes. Prolactin cells of transplantable rat pituitary tumors differ from "normal" prolactin cells in that they are not responsive to bromocriptine (85).

Inhibition of prolactin release in rats by bromocriptine can be counteracted dose-dependently by the dopamine receptor blocker chlorpromazine (39). *In vitro,* bromocriptine competes, as do apomorphine and dopamine, with [^{3}H]-dopamine (17) or [^{3}H]-dihydro-α-ergokryptine (21) for binding to anterior pituitary membranes *(see also Section VI, page 33)*. As hormone secretion from prolactin cells is under inhibitory dopamine control (96), it can be inferred that bromocriptine also inhibits prolactin release by stimulating dopamine receptors.

It is not known how stimulation of dopamine receptors on prolactin cells results in inhibition of hormone release. Prolactin release *in vitro* is increased by augmenting the available cAMP (81,118,124), and this effect can be antagonized by bromocriptine (119) or dopamine (81). Dopamine and bromocriptine were found to inhibit basal adenylate cyclase activity in rat pituitary homogenates (104) and in homogenates of human pituitary adenomas (33), but others have claimed that these drugs stimulate this enzyme in homogenates of rat, rabbit, and monkey anterior pituitaries (2,140) or do not produce any effect (140). Increasing $[K^+]$ in the incubating medium to 30 to 50 μM depolarizes the pituitary cell membranes (109), increases the Ca^{45}-space of rat pituitaries (108), and induces release of prolactin (54) without augmenting cAMP (178). This stimulated prolactin release is also inhibited by bromocriptine (54). As Ca^{2+} was found to be essential for mediating the actions of high $[K^+]$ and of TRH on prolactin release (159), and as bromocriptine antagonizes both stimulatory actions (39,54,139), it may be speculated that bromocriptine attenuates prolactin release by reducing the pool of intracellular free Ca^{2+} or by interfering with membrane functions.

B. Effects on Other Pituitary Hormones

1. Gonadotropins

Diverse actions of bromocriptine on gonadotropin secretion have been observed. These may or may not be related to the same basic property that is responsible for inhibition of prolactin secretion, i.e., dopamine-like activity. Since the neuronal control of gonadotropin secretion is still poorly understood, the discussion of drug effects in terms of receptor interactions remains highly speculative.

a. Induction of Secretion

Bromocriptine induces new ovarian cycles in pseudopregnant rats, regardless of whether this state was induced by implanting an ectopic source of prolactin (46) or by administering drugs that interfere with aminergic neuronal functions (45). Induction of phasic gonadotropin secretion is also observed in postpartum ewes treated with bromocriptine, but in normal cycling ewes the drug does not alter the ovarian cycle (76,77,121). In talapoin monkeys, socially subordinate females have elevated prolactin serum levels and the LH surge to an estrogen challenge is absent (11). When such monkeys were treated with bromocriptine, the prolactin level was lowered and an LH surge could be elicited. It is assumed that phasic gonadotropin secretion is restored in these species primarily as a consequence of the reduction of circulating prolactin levels, but in view of the dopaminergic involvement in gonadotropin control (71,82,88,106), bromocriptine may also have a direct action.

b. Inhibition of Secretion

Bromocriptine inhibits phasic gonadotropin secretion and ovulation in juvenile rats in which a premature cycle is induced by a booster dose of pregnant mare serum (53,71,100). We found that in such animals, inhibition of the preovulatory LH surge, and of ovulation, occurred in the same dose range as is necessary to suppress the preovulatory prolactin surge (100). In contrast, phasic gonadotropin secretion and ovulation in spontaneously cycling adult rats was only suppressed at much higher doses than are necessary to inhibit the preovulatory prolactin surge. Thus, it seems that in the juvenile rat, the neuronal control mechanism of phasic gonadotropin secretion is quite different from that in the adult rat. Adult female rats may be treated with bromocriptine for a prolonged period without interruption of cyclicity, but there is a time-dependent accumulation of nonfunctional corpora lutea due to repeated suppression of the (luteolytic) preovulatory prolactin surge (10). These facts should be considered when assessing the relative importance of dopamine in the control of LH secretion. A comparison of the ovulation inhibitory potency of a series of ergot compounds with their potency as inhibitors of implantation led to the conclusion that the two properties vary independently (43). This suggests that two qualitatively different mechanisms of action are responsible. LH surge suppression by such drugs in the adult rat could be due to serotonin antagonism (43,101,102). Bromocriptine has a low potency both as a serotonin antagonist *(see Section VI)* and as an inhibitor of spontaneous ovulation.

In adult male rats, prolonged treatment with prolactin-suppressing doses of bromocriptine did not change LH concentrations in the plasma or the pituitary (113).

2. *Somatotropin*

Bromocriptine does not seem to affect somatotropin (GH) secretion in experimental animals (153,171,173). In adult male rats treated with estrogens, bromocriptine did not influence the growth hormone response (32). Prolonged treatment with the drug did not alter serum GH levels in sheep (14), lactating goats (69), or cows (154), whereas in each instance prolactin was suppressed.

In cultures of rat pituitary cells (GH_3), bromocriptine did not alter basal GH release (158) or potassium-stimulated GH secretion (54) at drug concentrations that suppressed prolactin release. In contrast, bromocriptine was found to suppress GH as well as prolactin release in incubated adenoma tissue from acromegalic patients (74,105).

3. *Corticotropin*

There are no animal studies in which corticotropin (ACTH) was measured after bromocriptine treatment. Indirect evidence indicates that the drug probably has no relevant effects on ACTH secretion. In rats, after prolonged treatment with bromocriptine, no change in adrenal weight or plasma corticosterone level was found (19), and in lactating cows no effect on cortisol levels at milking was observed with doses of bromocriptine that effectively suppressed serum prolactin levels (154).

4. *Melanotropin*

Bromocriptine inhibits α-melanotropin (α-MSH) secretion in the rat (125,126). This is probably a direct action on the intermediate lobe of the pituitary, as α-MSH in the plasma is also suppressed in animals with lesions in the median eminence, which isolate the pituitary from hypothalamic control (126). In Syrian hamsters chronically treated with estrogens, bromocriptine attenuated the development of hyperplastic and neoplastic changes in the intermediate pituitary lobe (68).

5. *Thyrotropin*

No animal studies have been performed to assess the action of acute or prolonged treatment with bromocriptine on thyrotropin (TSH) secretion.

6. *Posterior Pituitary Hormones*

a. *Vasopressin*

In acute experiments in rats, bromocriptine did not influence water excretion (39), which indicates that vasopressin release was not altered by the drug. Prolonged treatment of rats with bromocriptine produced a fall in urine osmolality (98) and specific gravity (135), but it is not known whether this was due to a direct renal action of bromocriptine, to the suppression of prolactin, or to a slight inhibition of vasopressin secretion.

b. Oxytocin

Several ergot compounds (64–66) are known to suppress oxytocin release elicited by the suckling stimulus (milk ejection test) in lactating rats. Bromocriptine did not depress milk ejection (40). This is particularly interesting in view of the recent evidence, from *in vitro* studies (149), of an inhibitory dopaminergic mechanism regulating oxytocin release in rats.

C. Effects on Peripheral Endocrine Systems

1. Steroidogenic Organs

Various changes in steroidogenesis have been observed after bromocriptine administration. These were considered to be a consequence of the reduction of circulating prolactin rather than a direct effect of the drug. Thus, in the rat ovary, 20α-hydroxysteroid dehydrogenase activity increased after a single dose of bromocriptine injected on day 5, but not when given on day 16, of pregnancy; this effect could be counteracted by injecting prolactin (136). In the male mouse or rat, a reduction of circulating testosterone after prolonged treatment with bromocriptine has been reported (5,12). The role of prolactin in endocrine testicular functions is well recognized (6,7,67,147,148). Prolactin is involved in adrenal steroidogenesis of the rat (26,129,169,170).

2. Other Systems

It is known that dopamine stimulates cAMP formation in parathyroid gland cells *in vitro* and increases parathyroid hormone release (13). However, sensitivity of parathyroid gland cells to dopamine is considered to be transmitted via D-1 receptors, which are distinguished from the D-2 receptors of prolactin cells by being linked to adenylate cyclase (78). No information is available concerning an action of bromocriptine on parathyroid cells. Renin release in dogs (73) as well as insulin and glucagon secretion in man (86,94) were also observed to be stimulated by dopamine infusion. Again, no experimental data concerning an effect of bromocriptine on the secretion of these hormones are available.

III. CNS ACTIONS

Bromocriptine has a number of actions in extra-hypophyseotropic areas of the brain. Some of these effects can be observed with doses similar to those needed to inhibit prolactin secretion in the same species, whereas other central effects occur only at higher doses.

A. Autonomic Functions

Bromocriptine is a powerful emetic in the dog, the ED_{50} being 7.5 μg/kg i.v. and 11.4 μg/kg s.c., respectively. By the i.v. route, bromocriptine was approximately three times less emetic than its parent compound, α-ergokryptine, and 2.5 times less active than ergotamine.

Bromocriptine lowers body temperature in rats exposed to a cold environment, and this can be prevented by the dopamine antagonists pimozide (18), haloperidol, and sulpiride (72*a*). It is concluded that this is a dopamine-like action in the thermoregulatory regions of the brain. In mice pretreated with reserpine to induce hypothermia, bromocriptine raised the body temperature; this effect could be prevented by sulpiride (72). In rabbits, a rise in body temperature was observed after bromocriptine administration (92,99). Haloperidol prevented the hyperthermia caused by a low dose of bromocriptine, but had no effect on the hyperthermic action of a high dose. Cyproheptadine blocked the hyperthermic action of a low and of a high dose (99), which suggests that bromocriptine, besides having a dopamine-like action, also elicits central serotonin-like effects.

B. Locomotor Activity

Bromocriptine exerts a biphasic effect on motor activity in small rodents (75). In the first hour after s.c. administration to unaccustomed mice, a reduction in exploratory activity can be observed. Apomorphine and L-DOPA induce a similar initial depression, whereas *d*-amphetamine, a drug that facilitates the release of endogenous catecholamines, increases exploratory activity. Following the initial depression, bromocriptine, like L-DOPA and *d*-amphetamine, elicits strong locomotor stimulation, lasting from the second to the fifth hour. By analogy to the standard drug, it is assumed that the effects of bromocriptine on locomotor activity depend on catecholaminergic mechanisms. It has been suggested (34,156), as was previously done for apomorphine (20), that the initial depression induced by bromocriptine is due to a stimulant effect of low doses on (presynaptic) autoreceptors, i.e., on inhibitory dopamine receptors situated on the endings of dopaminergic neurons. This explanation of the biphasic behavioral effect of bromocriptine is not supported by biochemical data: in mice and rats, bromocriptine (156) and apomorphine (20) do not elicit biphasic alterations in dopamine metabolism in the central nervous system. A reduced turnover of dopamine is observed during both the initial depression and the subsequent increase in locomotor activity. Experimental evidence for autoreceptor interactions of bromocriptine will be given below.

When bromocriptine (128) or apomorphine (29) is administered bilaterally into the nucleus accumbens of rats, no motor stimulation is seen. However, immediately after injection, both drugs reduce dopamine-induced hyperactivity. Bromocriptine and apomorphine seem to be without agonist action on those receptors in the nucleus accumbens that are stimulated by dopamine but appear instead to act as antagonists.

C. Stereotypies

Bromocriptine, like apomorphine, *d*-amphetamine, and L-DOPA, induces stereotyped behavior in rodents (75). This consists of repetitive sniffing, gnawing, and biting. Stereotyped behavior elicited by bromocriptine appears to depend on dopamine receptor stimulation, since it is inhibited by pimozide (75), a selective blocker of dopamine receptors (3). Since bromocriptine-induced stereotypies were prevented by inhibiting catecholamine synthesis with α-methyl-p-tyrosine or by depleting catecholamine stores with reserpine, bromocriptine was thought to act indirectly (75). Others (132), observing only weak inhibition of bromocriptine-induced stereotypy by α-methyl-p-tyrosine, and even potentiation by reserpine, concluded that bromocriptine is a direct dopamine receptor agonist. The inhibitory effect of α-methyl-p-tyrosine may be explained by a nonspecific central depression, which masks the moderate stimulatory effect of bromocriptine.

In guinea pigs given prolonged treatment with bromocriptine at a daily dose that did not elicit stereotyped behavior, the sensitivity of the animals was found to increase with time if a challenging dose of *d*-amphetamine or apomorphine was given (120). This hypersensitivity persisted for several weeks after cessation of daily bromocriptine treatment. In rats, an increased sensitivity was already evident on the day following the first treatment with a centrally effective dose of bromocriptine (166).

D. Reserpine Antagonism

Central dopamine receptor agonists are potent inhibitors of the behavioral depression induced by depletion of catecholamine stores. Bromocriptine, like apomorphine, reduced the akinesia in mice caused by the previous administration of reserpine (174). In rats, akinesia induced by tetrabenazine (47) or perchlorperazine (132) was also inhibited by bromocriptine. Further, in rats treated with a high i.v. dose of reserpine to induce a state of α-rigidity, bromocriptine, like apomorphine and L-DOPA, was found to interrupt this state (Vigouret, J. M., *unpublished observation*).

E. Effects in Animals with Brain Lesions

Unilateral administration of small amounts of 6-hydroxy-dopamine into the zona compacta of the substantia nigra of the rat results in selective degeneration of the dopaminergic nigro-striatal pathways on the treated side (163). In such animals, dopamine receptor agonists such as apomorphine induce circling movements away from the lesioned side (contralateral rotations), whereas indirectly acting drugs such as *d*-amphetamine induce ipsilateral rotations (28,75). The effect of bromocriptine in such rats is similar to that of apomorphine. Contralateral turning induced by bromocriptine is inferred to be due to a stimulant effect on post-synaptic dopamine receptors in the striatum of the lesioned side, which, owing to degeneration of their presynaptic inputs, have developed denervation supersensitivity (163). However, bromocriptine-induced contralateral turning was blocked not only by pimozide, but also by α-methyl-p-tyrosine (93), this latter effect possibly being due to nonspecific depression.

Unilateral electrolytic lesions in the ventromedial tegmentum of the brain stem of Green monkeys induce hypokynesia and tremors, which can be counteracted by dopamine receptor agonists (57). Bromocriptine treatment results in reduced tremor intensity and initial sedation. The effect of bromocriptine lasts longer than that of L-DOPA, and pretreatment with haloperidol or α-methyl-p-tyrosine reduces the antitremor effect of bromocriptine (110).

F. Neurobiochemistry

Fluorescence microscopy studies by Hökfelt and Fuxe (71) first suggested that bromocriptine reduced transmitter turnover in central dopaminergic neurons. Corrodi et al. (28) confirmed this interpretation biochemically, showing in bromocriptine-treated rats a moderate elevation of brain dopamine content and reduced depletion of brain dopamine after inhibition of its synthesis. The authors concluded that bromocriptine is a direct stimulator of neuronal dopamine receptors. They also found a decrease in brain norepinephrine content and enhanced depletion of this amine after synthesis inhibition. Other investigators (16,103,165) have also described a moderate increase in dopamine content together with a long-lasting reduction of DOPAC in brain tissue, as well as an increase in MOPEG-SO_4, a metabolite of norepinephrine. In addition, they observed an increase in the levels of serotonin and 5-HIAA in the cerebral cortex. No change of serotonin and 5-HIAA levels was reported by some laboratories (27), whereas others (156) observed an increase in serotonin and a reduction of 5-HIAA in the brain. These authors pointed out that bromocriptine possibly reduced serotonin release directly by an effect on serotoninergic neurons, or indirectly by a dopaminomimetic action.

Recently, it was claimed that bromocriptine inhibits monoamine oxidase in the hypothalamus and liver of the rat (155), but such a property could not be found with the enzyme isolated from the whole brain (15). In view of the observed increase in brain MOPEG-SO_4, inhibition of monoamine oxidase activity appears to be a rather unlikely property of the drug.

It was observed that bromocriptine decreased and then increased acetylcholine release from the cerebral cortex of anesthetized rats (127). After apomorphine administration only, acetylcholine output was stimulated. Chronic septal lesions suppressed the stimulation but left the inhibitory effect of bromocriptine unchanged. The stimulatory effect of both drugs was suppressed by pretreatment with haloperidol, indicating that this effect is probably elicited directly through a dopaminergic system (111).

Recently, changes in brain transition-metal concentrations were reported to occur in guinea pigs after prolonged daily treatment with a combination of L-DOPA plus carbidopa or other centrally acting dopaminomimetic agents (167). After bromocriptine was given, the manganese concentration increased in the caudate nucleus, the frontal cortex, and the cerebellar hemispheres. Copper concentration decreased in these same areas, whereas iron decreased in the frontal cortex, remained unchanged in the caudate nucleus, and increased in the cerebellum. The authors believed that these effects were connected with the development of supersensitivity to dopaminomimetic compounds (120) and with the development in the clinic of psychosis and abnormal movements

(167) after long-term therapy of parkinsonian patients with dopaminomimetic drugs.

IV. CARDIOVASCULAR ACTIONS

A. Experiments in Cats

Bromocriptine was infused i.v., in increasing concentrations up to 18.7 mg/kg, in cats anesthetized with chloralose-urethane (39). Following administration of 0.1 mg/kg or more, decreases of both blood pressure and heart rate were observed that were not clearly dose-dependent. An intracerebro-ventricular injection of 10 μg/kg—which had little effect when given intravenously—produced bradycardia and a reduction of blood pressure of about 30 mmHg, which persisted for about 2 hr. This indicates that bromocriptine exerts an inhibitory effect on vasomotor centers.

In the pithed cat, bromocriptine attenuated transmission in the cardiac sympathetic nerves at doses from 10 μg/kg i.v. and higher. Significant inhibition of heart rate increases occurred in response to both pre- and postganglionic nerve stimulation. This effect was inhibited in a dose-dependent manner by haloperidol but not by the serotonin receptor blocker pizotifen, nor by the α-adrenoceptor antagonist phentolamine (24,143). These results are interpreted as indicating stimulation by bromocriptine of prejunctional dopamine receptors on the sympathetic nerve endings, as is also seen after apomorphine administration (142). These receptors, when activated, reduce the quanta of norepinephrine released per nerve impulse (133). Similar findings were recently obtained with the perfused central artery of the rabbit ear (177).

B. Experiments in Dogs

Bromocriptine lowered blood pressure and decreased resistance in the superior mesenteric vascular bed in chloralose-urethane anesthetized dogs (24,39). This action was dose dependent from 6 μg/kg i.v. and lasted for more than 2 hr. Reflex tachycardia was rarely seen. Both effects could be abolished by pretreating the animal with haloperidol, ergometrine, or methyl-ergometrine, which are selective dopamine receptor blocking agents in blood vessels (8,23,174). Further evidence for such an action of bromocriptine on vascular dopamine receptors was derived from experiments where the celiac, superior and inferior mesenteric, and renal arteries—vascular beds considered to contain dopamine receptors (35)—were excluded from the circulation by tying them off. In such a preparation, using barbiturate anesthesia, bromocriptine did not lower blood pressure (23).

The experiments in cats and dogs suggest three possible sites of action for the hypotensive effects of bromocriptine: CNS, sympathetic nerve terminal, and vascular smooth muscle. At each putative site of action the effect of bromocriptine might be due to stimulation of dopamine receptors. The relative importance, in the intact organism, of these three sites of action is still unknown.

C. Experiments in the Pithed Rat

Bromocriptine, when injected intravenously into pithed rats, induced small, dose-dependent increases of blood pressure. This vasopressor effect was found to be about 50 times less than that of the parent compound α-ergokryptine, which in turn was two to five times less potent than ergotamine (157).

V. MISCELLANEOUS ACTIONS

A. Effects on the Uterus

Bromocriptine, unlike either its parent compound α-ergokryptine or ergotamine and methylergometrine, did not have oxytocic activity on the uterus of anesthetized rabbits studied *in situ* when given in doses up to 0.5 mg/kg i.v. Instead, it inhibited the uterine response to methylergometrine (157). The action of bromocriptine on the rabbit uterus thus resembles that of dihydrogenated ergopeptides (138).

B. Effects on the Intestine

Bromocriptine decreased intestinal propulsion of charcoal in mice with an ED_{50} of 20 mg/kg s.c. (39). This is a very high dose compared to that needed to inhibit prolactin secretion or cause dopaminergic effects at the CNS level. Atropine was similarly active in reducing intestinal propulsion (ED_{50} = 19 mg/kg s.c.), whereas apomorphine was somewhat less potent (ED_{50} = 34 mg/kg s.c.). The effect was observed only in acute experiments. After administration of 32 mg/kg s.c. on 4 consecutive days, the fifth dose of bromocriptine did not slow the propulsion of charcoal. Thus, tolerance to the gastrointestinal inhibitory effect quickly developed.

C. Effects on Renal Function

Bromocriptine, given to rats as a single oral dose (10 mg/kg) or a single s.c. dose (1 mg/kg), produced no consistent changes in water or electrolyte excretion in our laboratory (39). Others have described a reduction in sodium, potassium, and calcium excretion after higher single doses (97). When given over several days to rats, the compound was found to increase urine volume as well as sodium, potassium, and calcium output (98). During prolonged oral administration of high doses of bromocriptine, the composition of the urine of treated rats differed from that of controls after 6, 13, 26, and 52 weeks: increased excretory values for sodium, potassium, and water per 24 hr were observed (135), together with an increased urinary pH and a decreased specific gravity and calcium excretion. Of particular interest was the finding that the kidneys of the treated animals showed a lower incidence and a decreased severity of the spontaneous degenerative lesions usually encountered in this species. In anesthetized dogs given single i.v. doses of bromocriptine, no dose-dependent changes in renal plasma flow, glomerular filtration rate, or electrolyte and water excretion were found with doses up to 0.3 mg/kg i.v. (39).

VI. RECEPTOR INTERACTIONS

A. Experiments Involving α-Adrenoceptors, Serotonin Receptors, and Cholinergic Receptors

Bromocriptine, as an ergot peptide derivative, is expected to show affinity to α-adrenoceptors and serotonin receptors (117). To assess these properties *in vitro,* spiral strips of femoral veins and basilar arteries from mongrel dogs (115,116) and the perfused mesenteric artery of the rat (55) were used. On canine venous strips, bromocriptine developed only negligible stimulatory (intrinsic) activity but inhibited the action of norepinephrine competitively ($pA_2 = 8.9$), being about three times less potent than dihydroergotamine. In the rat mesenteric artery, on the other hand, norepinephrine was antagonized in a noncompetitive way ($pD'_2 = 8.5$). On canine arterial strips, bromocriptine showed only negligible stimulatory activity but antagonized the action of serotonin noncompetitively ($pD'_2 = 7.6$), being about 30 times less potent than dihydroergotamine. Although ergot compounds are not known to interact with acetylcholine receptors (117), bromocriptine, in view of its inhibitory action on gastrointestinal motility in mice, was tested in the guinea pig ileum (39). In concentrations up to $10^{-3.9}$M, it neither contracted nor relaxed the isolated ileum. It inhibited responses to added acetylcholine, this antagonistic action of bromocriptine being of the noncompetitive type and occurring only at concentrations several orders of magnitude higher ($pD'_2 = 5.1$) than those required to produce the classic actions at α-adrenoceptors and serotonin receptors.

B. Experiments Involving Dopamine Receptors

In several of the experiments described, bromocriptine was found to act like dopamine, i.e., to be a dopaminomimetic agent. More direct evidence for interaction with dopamine receptors was obtained by studying isolated dopamine sensitive preparations.

1. Dopamine-Sensitive Adenylate Cyclase

When given systemically to rats, bromocriptine, like apomorphine, increased cAMP in the striatum (161,162) but not in the hypothalamus (130). However, when added to a dopamine-sensitive adenylate system in rat brain homogenates, bromocriptine—in contrast to dopamine and apomorphine—did not stimulate (103,161,162), or stimulated to only a small extent (52), the production of cAMP. When added together with dopamine to this enzyme preparation, bromocriptine antagonized the stimulatory effect of dopamine in a dose-dependent manner.

From such experiments (103) using slices or homogenates of rat striatum, the affinity of bromocriptine to the dopamine receptor was calculated ($pA_2 = 6.9$ for slices; $pA_2 = 6.1$ for homogenates). In isolated rabbit retinae, bromocriptine, at high concentrations, was found to stimulate cAMP production, like dopamine and similarly acting agents (144). Other studies, using pituitary tissue, have produced conflicting results. Dopamine and related drugs, at 10^{-5}M, did not influence cAMP concentration in dispersed rat anterior pituitary cells (112) or in pituitary homogenates (140). In a more recent study, dopamine and bromocriptine, at concentrations from 10^{-7} to 10^{-5}M, were both found to lower cAMP concentrations in rat anterior pituitary homogenates (104), which is compatible with the observation that dopamine and related agents depress cAMP formation in homogenates of human pituitary adenoma tissue (33). In contrast, other investigators found stimulation of cAMP formation when dopamine, bromocriptine, and similar drugs were incubated with homogenates of anterior pituitaries of rat and monkey (2). This latter result is also in conflict with the observation that prolactin release *in vitro* is augmented by increasing the available cAMP (81,118,124), which effect can be antagonized by bromocriptine (119) or dopamine (81). Thus, the data do not establish clearly whether or not the receptor involved in prolactin secretion inhibition is linked to an adenylate cyclase.

2. Receptor Binding Studies

Using membranes isolated from bovine anterior pituitaries, bromocriptine was found to compete at a low concentration (10^{-8}M) with the specific binding of [^{3}H]-dopamine (17). Bromocriptine competed with the specific binding of [^{3}H]-dihydro-α-ergokryptine to DA receptors of such membranes with a K_D of 24 nmoles, being about 20 times more potent than dopamine, or three times more potent than apomorphine (21). With sheep anterior pituitary membranes using [^{3}H]-spiroperidol as the ligand (31), bromocriptine competed with its binding with a K_I of 18.5 nmoles, being about 70 times more potent than dopamine and about 12 times more potent than apomorphine. In another study with bovine anterior pituitary membranes, bromocriptine competed with the binding of [^{3}H]-spiroperidol with a K_I of 3.1 nmoles, being 3,000 times more potent than dopamine and 100 times more active than apomorphine (30). Thus, with anterior pituitary membranes, bromocriptine showed a similar high activity when competing with a dopamine receptor agonist (dihydro-α-ergokryptine) and an antagonist (spiroperidol).

Similar studies were also conducted using membranes of brain origin. Bromocriptine competed with the binding of [^{3}H]-dopamine and [^{3}H]-apomorphine to rat striatal membranes with a K_I of 76 and 16.4 nmoles, respectively (57), and with [^{3}H]-dopamine binding to bovine striatal membranes with a K_I of 300 nmoles (56,87). When antagonists—instead of dopamine receptor agonists—were used as ligands, bromocriptine was more potent: it competed with the binding of [^{3}H]-haloperidol or [^{3}H]-spiroperidol with a K_I of 7.8 and 1.75 nmoles, respectively (57). Using [^{3}H]-spiroperidol as the ligand to membranes of bovine caudate nucleus (30), bromocriptine competed with a K_I of 3.5 nmoles, being 1,000 times more potent than dopamine and 40 times more active than apomorphine. These results indicate that with membranes derived from various brain areas, bromocriptine seems to compete more actively with the binding of dopamine antagonists than of dopamine agonists.

The binding studies support the idea that in the brain, two different binding sites for dopamine are present (160); the results show that bromocriptine has a higher affinity for the "antagonist" binding site than for the "agonist" binding site. On pituitary-derived membranes, no such distinction is apparent. The affinity of bromocriptine for binding sites on pituitary membranes is very similar to its affinity for "antagonist" sites on membranes derived from the brain.

VII. TOXICITY IN ANIMALS

A. Acute Studies

The effects of a single oral or intravenous dose of bromocriptine mesylate were studied in mice, rats, and rabbits (59). Observations were made of the signs before death, those elicited by the maximal tolerated dose, the time of death, and the overall mortality for a period of 7 days. When death was the result, it occurred within 24 hr after drug administration. Necropsy was performed on all animals, but no specific drug-induced effects were revealed. In rats and rabbits, no deaths occurred at the highest doses that could be administered orally. The LD_{50} values obtained are given in Table 1. Following i.v. administration, initial signs of toxicity

TABLE 1. *24-hr LD_{50} values for bromocriptine mesylate*

	LD_{50} mg/kg ± standard deviation	
	Intravenous	Oral
Mouse	190 ± 9.3	2,620 ± 604[a]
Rat	72 ± 3.5	>2,000[b]
Rabbit	12.5 ± 3.6	>1,000[b]

[a] Extrapolated.
[b] The highest dose that could be administered; no deaths.

were dyspnea and motor excitation, gradually leading to rhythmic cramps, slowing of respiration, and coma. Similar signs occurred after oral administration, but their sequence was less rapid.

B. Prolonged Studies

1. Rats (a)

The effects of repeated daily oral administration of bromocriptine were studied over 53 weeks in male and female rats (60). Four groups received either unmedicated feed or feed containing bromocriptine to yield mean doses of 5, 20, and 82 mg/kg/day. Additional rats were examined at the mid- and high-dose levels after a further 5-week "recovery" period with unmedicated feed. A dose of 5 mg/kg/day was associated with slightly increased weight gain in males and decreased weight gain in females. Post-mortem studies revealed slightly increased adrenal weights and decreased pituitary weights in females. An increase in cystic ovarian follicles associated with decreased luteal tissue and squamous metaplasia of the endometrium suggested an endocrine effect at this dosage. There was a lower incidence and severity of chronic, progressive nephropathy in males as compared to controls, which may be attributed to prolactin inhibition (135).

Twenty mg/kg/day caused slight excitability at intervals, the same effects on weight gain as seen with 5 mg/kg/day and, in 2 of 30 rats, blue discoloration of the tail tip, first seen after 37 weeks of treatment. Adrenal weights were increased and pituitary weights decreased in females. All females had increased numbers of abnormal corpora lutea and cystic follicles of the ovaries, associated with pyometra or endometritis, suggesting estrogen dominance. Again, at this dose level there was an apparent improvement in interstitial nephritis.

At 82 mg/kg/day, there were similar but more pronounced changes to those seen at the lower doses. In addition, epileptiform convulsions on handling occurred after 45 weeks of drug administration. There was a slight trend toward reduced leukocyte counts, but all individual values were within normal limits and differential counts revealed no deviations from normal. Examination of the "recovery" rats, after a 5-week drug-free period, revealed almost complete reversal of morphologic changes, and a return to the level of changes expected in 65-week-old rats.

The presence of cystic follicles and corresponding estrogen-induced endometrial changes were not predictable on the basis of the selective prolactin-inhibiting action that bromocriptine possesses. Basic knowledge of the actions of bromocriptine is derived from studies in animals with fully active endocrine systems. The findings in this prolonged experiment must therefore be considered against a background of a spontaneously declining endocrine activity (the presence of follicular cysts and endometrial hyperplasia in some control rats indicated that this was the case). The effects on the female sex organs and the kidneys were regarded as pharmacodynamic rather than toxic in nature. Toxicity at the high dosage was expressed by cyanosis of the tail tip and CNS signs—both known effects of overdosage of ergot derivatives.

2. Rats (b)

Four groups of male and female rats were given bromocriptine in the feed for 100 weeks (62). Drug concentrations were chosen to provide mean daily intakes of 0, 1.7, 9.8, and 44 mg/kg.

At low doses, there was a reduction in the incidence and severity of periarteritis (a known age-related process in rats), an increased incidence of inflammatory, hyperplastic, and metaplastic changes in the uterus, and a significant reduction in the total number of tumors in females as shown in Table 2.

At the mid- and high-dose levels, there was a significant decrease in the mortality of males due to delayed onset and decreased severity of chronic progressive nephropathy (135), another age-related disease of rats. In females, inflammatory, hyperplastic, metaplastic, and neoplastic changes were seen in the uterus. There was a significant decrease in the overall number of tumors in females at both doses (fewer mammary tumors), and in males at high doses (fewer adrenal tumors). On the other hand, the incidence of uterine neoplasia was increased, as shown in the Table 2.

Most of the effects listed above can be regarded as beneficial. However, the increase in uterine tumors clearly required further investigation. A series of additional experiments showed that as the female rats age, the cyclicity of reproductive events deteriorates and prolonged periods of pseudopregnancy alternate with persistent estrus. The spontaneous occurrence, in aging rats, of these prolonged phases of estrus or of pseudopregnancy has been observed by others (4,107) and was shown to be due to hypothalamic, and not ovarian, failure.

Bromocriptine, owing to its prolactin-suppressing action, prevented the occurrence of pseudopregnancy and correspondingly increased the incidence and duration of the alternative situation in aging rats—persistent estrus. Plasma estradiol and progesterone levels in rats from the 100-week study showed that bromocriptine administration inhibited the rise in progesterone levels associated with the state of pseudopregnancy, although basal progesterone levels were unaffected. There was no evidence of a drug effect on estradiol levels in rats at any time during the study, or on the progesterone levels in young female rats, i.e., rats examined early in the study. Progesterone-estradiol ratios correlated well with uterine histology, low ratios being associated with endometrial metaplasia or uterine neoplasia. The findings indicate that the observed endometrial changes in the bromocriptine-treated rats are a consequence of the long periods of uninterrupted estrogen stimulation to which these aging females were exposed. Similar endometrial changes have been observed in rats with constant estrus, e.g., after neonatal masculinization (25,58).

3. Dogs

Bromocriptine was given orally once daily for 62 weeks to adult male and female beagles (63). Because of emesis the initial doses were small, but they were escalated over the first 10 weeks,

TABLE 2. *Deaths and tumors in rats given bromocriptine in their food for 100 weeks*

	Controls		Low-dose		Mid-dose		High-dose	
	Male	Female	Male	Female	Male	Female	Male	Female
Rats in study	50	50	50	50	50	50	50	50
Death by 100 weeks	36	32	28	25	21[a]	24	19[a]	32
Rats with tumors	28	44	30	29[a]	28	26[a]	19	20[a]
Benign mammary tumors	—	37	—	14[a]	—	10[a]	—	8[a]
Malignant mammary tumors	—	3	—	1	—	0	—	0
Benign adrenal tumors	19	2	12	2	14	1	3[a]	1
Benign uterine tumors	—	0	—	0	—	1	—	0
Malignant uterine tumors	—	0	—	2	—	7[a]	—	9[a]

[a] $p < 0.01$ vs control group (one-sided Fisher's exact test).

so that for the following 52 weeks the daily doses were 1, 3, and 10 mg/kg. Four dogs were examined after an additional 8-week period without drug treatment.

During the period of increasing doses, the following symptoms were observed: excess salivation, impaired food intake and weight gain (weight loss in some dogs), slightly decreased hemoglobin values, and mild functional ECG changes. Vomiting in this period was intense immediately after each increase in dose, and the above findings were considered to be secondary to this.

The following effects emerged or persisted in all treated dogs, irrespective of final dosage, during the following year: slight mydriasis in weeks 1 to 4, and slight sedation, prolapse of the nictitating membranes, and sporadic dacryorrhea throughout the study. Other effects observed in some of the treated dogs are listed together with their incidence in Table 3. Melanosis, impaired hair growth, and necrosis of ear margins occurred earlier in the high-dose animals than in other groups. With 10 mg/kg, additional nonspecific pathology was seen: hepatocyte swelling and occasional degeneration, mild degenerative lesions of the gastric mucosa, hypertrophy of the adrenal cortex, and atrophy of Peyer's patches. No specific toxic effect emerged. Examination of the "recovery" dogs showed that with the exception of melanosis

TABLE 3. *Prolonged oral administration of bromocriptine in dogs*

	No. of dogs affected		
	Dosage		
Effect	1 mg/kg	3 mg/kg	10 mg/kg
Melanosis of sexual skin	6/6	4/6	3/6
Alopecia	1/6	1/6	1/6
Cystic ovarian follicles	2/3	2/3	2/3
Cystic corpora lutea	3/3	2/3	2/3
Thyroid hyperactivity	3/6	3/6	3/6
Increased pituitary eosinophils	0/6	1/6	4/6
Necrosis of ear margins	0/6	2/6	5/6

and alopecia in 1 of 4 dogs, all pathological findings were fully reversible within 8 weeks.

Apart from the early effects, which were secondary to intense vomiting, all changes were regarded as expressions of exaggerated pharmacodynamic activity or nonspecific effects of overdosage. Not unexpectedly, prolonged administration caused some endocrine effects. Increased melanin deposition in the sexual skin accompanies hormonal imbalance in dogs (114). The ovarian changes suggest a drug effect on the female endocrine system; corresponding changes were not seen in male gonads. Bilateral alopecia and inhibition of hair growth (observed at the shaved ECG recording sites) may be related to the prolactin-inhibiting effect, as this hormone may be an important factor in hair growth in the dog (134). The microscopic changes in the anterior pituitary and thyroid suggest possible drug-related effects on these organs. Superficial epithelial necrosis of dependent ear margins is characteristic of overdosage with ergot alkaloids in dogs with low-hanging ears and represents a trophic response to an effect on the vasculature at an extremely sensitive site.

4. Rhesus Monkeys

Bromocriptine was given once daily by stomach tube (as a suspension in tragacanth) to three groups of adult male and female rhesus monkeys, at doses of 2, 8, and 32 mg/kg, for 13 weeks (61). Positive effects, which could be related to treatment, are summarized in Table 4. As can be seen, no specific toxic effects of bromocriptine medication emerged. Excitability was transient at the low-dose level. Weight loss was seen in the early weeks, both in controls and treated animals, and was probably caused by the initial stress of oral intubation. Decreased splenic weights occurred in treated monkeys, but this was not accompanied by any pathologic changes and presumably represented an expression of a functional drug effect. Slight anemia occurred in 1 monkey after 13 weeks at the high-dose level. Histologically, some swelling of basophil cells in the anterior pituitary was noted in 2 monkeys

TABLE 4. *Effects of 13 weeks of oral bromocriptine in rhesus monkeys*

Effect	Dosage			
	0 (Controls)	2 mg/kg/day	8 mg/kg/day	32 mg/kg/day
Excitability	−	+	+	+
Initial weight loss	+	+	+	++
Continued weight loss	−	−	−	+
Anemia (incidence)	−	−	−	+
Decreased spleen weight	−	+	+	++

Note: − Absent; + weakly present; ++ obvious.

at the high-dose level. This finding contrasts with that in dogs following bromocriptine administration for 1 year, where an increase in the number of pituitary eosinophils (see Table 3) was seen with doses ranging from 1 to 10 mg/kg/day (63). The discrepancy may be related to the different doses at which the effects were seen.

VIII. PHARMACOKINETICS AND METABOLIC FATE

Bromocriptine, as well as most other ergot derivatives, poses great analytic problems for biopharmaceutical studies. These are due partly to the low doses used therapeutically and partly to the physicochemical properties and the metabolic fate of these compounds. Ergopeptides and their derivatives, e.g., bromocriptine, further complicate biopharmaceutical work, in that only a small fraction of an administered dose is excreted in the urine, the main excretory route (>90%) being the bile and feces (36,80).

A. Rats

Using both a RIA system, which was highly sensitive to structural features of the peptide moiety of ergopeptines, and radiolabeled bromocriptine (145), an oral bioavailability of only 6% was found, together with a high hepatic extraction rate. In the pituitary, bromocriptine reached high concentrations. Comparison of pharmacokinetic parameters of bromocriptine with its hypothermic effect (18) suggest that this dopaminomimetic effect is due to the intact molecule (48,79) and not to metabolites, as has been suggested (152).

B. Man

1. In healthy subjects, comparison of acute oral versus intravenous pharmacokinetics showed a nearly complete absorbtion of ^{3}H-labeled bromocriptine (1) from the gastrointestinal tract, with a maximal plasma level at about 1.4 hr. The urinary excretion reached only about 6% of the dose in 96 hr. This is typical for ergopeptines (36).

2. Using the same RIA system as in the rat study mentioned above, together with C^{14}-labeled bromocriptine, pharmacokinetic studies have been performed in normal subjects and hyperprolactinemic female patients (146). In an oral dose range of 1 to 7.5 mg, a strong correlation between dose and the peak plasma level or the area under the plasma concentration curve (ng/liter × hr) was found. Compartmental analysis of the data gave results consistent with incomplete oral absorption and "first pass" metabolism of the drug. Bromocriptine levels in hyperprolactinemic patients after 3 and 6 months of bromocriptine treatment (2.5 mg t.i.d. at 6-hr intervals) were found to agree with multiple dose projections from single dose parameters.

3. In parkinsonian patients given single doses of 12.5, 25, 50, or 100 mg bromocriptine orally (131), plasma bromocriptine concentrations obtained by RIA showed considerable interindividual variation. After 50 and 100 mg, plasma levels were still high after 4 hr. No significant correlation was found between peak plasma levels and peak clinical response, maximal increase of growth hormone, or reduction in blood pressure. Peak biological effects followed shortly after peak plasma drug levels.

4. In a further study of patients with Parkinson's disease, using steady state conditions (50) and a gas chromatographic method to measure plasma levels of intact bromocriptine, excellent correlation between the oral dose and the area under the individual plasma concentration curve (ng/liter × hr) was found.

REFERENCES

1. Aellig, W. H., and Nüesch, E. (1977): Comparative pharmokinetic investigations with tritium-labelled ergot alkaloids after oral and intravenous administration in man. *Int. J. Clin. Pharmacol.,* 15:106–112.
2. Ahn, H. S., Gardner, E., and Makman, M. H. (1978): Anterior pituitary adenylate cyclase: Stimulation by dopamine and other monoamines. *Eur. J. Pharmacol.,* 53:313–317.
3. Andén, N. E., Butcher, S. G., Corrodi, H., Fuxe, K., and Ungerstedt, U. (1970): Receptor activity and turnover of dopamine and noradrenaline after neuroleptics. *Eur. J. Pharmacol.,* 11:303–314.
4. Aschheim, P. (1965): La réaction de l'ovaire des rattes séniles en oestrus permanent au moyen d'hormones gonadotropes ou de la mise à l'obscurité. *C. R. Acad. Sci., (Paris),* 260:2627–2630.
5. Bartke, A. (1973): Plasma testosterone levels in male mice and rats treated with inhibitors of prolactin release. *Acta Endocrinol., (Khb.),* 177(Suppl.):22.
6. Bartke, A. (1974): Effects of inhibitors of pituitary prolactin release on testicular cholesterol stores, seminal vesicles weight, fertility and lactation in mice. *Biol. Reprod.,* 11:319–325.
7. Bartke, A., and Dalterio, S. (1976): Effects of prolactin on the sensitivity of the testis to LH. *Biol. Reprod.,* 15:90–93.
8. Bell, C., Convay, E. L., and Lang, W. J. (1974): Ergometrine and apomorphine as selective antagonists of dopamine in the canine renal vasculature. *Br. J. Pharmacol.,* 52:591–599.
9. Berde, B., and Stürmer, E. (1978): Introduction to the pharmacology of ergot alkaloids and related compounds as a basis of their therapeutic application. In: *Ergot Alkaloids and Related Compounds. Handbook of Experimental Pharmacology, Vol. 49,* edited by B. Berde and H. O. Schild, pp. 1–28. Springer Verlag, Heidelberg.
10. Billeter, E., and Flückiger, E. (1971): Evidence for a luteolytic function of prolactin in the intact cyclic rat using 2-Br-α-ergokryptine (CB 154). *Experientia,* 27:464–465.
11. Bowman, L., Dilley, S., and Keverne, E. B. (1978): Suppression of oestrogen-induced LH surges by social subordination in talapoin monkey. *Nature,* 275:56–58.
12. Boyns, A. R., Cole, E. N., Golder, M. P., Danutra, V., Harper, M. E., Brownsey, B., Cowley, T., Jones, G. E., and Griffiths, K. (1972): Prolactin

studies with the prostate. Tenovus Workshop. In: *Prolactin and Carcinogenesis,* edited by A. R. Boyns and K. Griffiths, pp. 207–216. Alpha Omega Alpha Publishing, Cardiff, U.K.

13. Brown, E. M., Carroll, R. J., and Aurbach, G. D. (1977): Dopaminergic stimulation of cyclic AMP accumulation and parathyroid hormone release from dispersed bovine parathyroid cells. *Biochemistry,* 74:4210–4213.
14. Brown, W. B., Driver, P. M., Jones, R., and Forbes, J. M. (1976): Growth, prolactin and growth hormone in lambs treated with CB 154. *J. Endocrinol.,* 69:47P.
15. Bürki, H. R. (1978): Lack of effect of bromocriptine on the activity of monoamine oxydase in rat brain. *J. Pharm. Pharmacol,.* 30:261.
16. Bürki, H. R., Asper, H., Ruch, W., and Züger, P. E. (1978): Bromocriptine, dihydroergotoxine, methysergide, *d*-LSD, CF 25–397, and 29–712: Effects on the metabolism of the biogenic amines in the brain of the rat. *Psychopharmacology,* 57:227–237.
17. Calabro, M. A., and MacLeod, R. M. (1978): Binding of dopamine to bovine anterior pituitary gland membranes. *Neuroendocrinology,* 25:32–46.
18. Calne, D. B., Claveria, L. E., and Reid, J. C. (1975): Hypothermic action of bromocriptine. *Br. J. Pharmacol.,* 54:123–124.
19. Cameron, E. H. D., and Scarisbrick, J. J. (1973): Determination of corticosterone in rat plasma by competitive protein-binding assay and its use in assessing the effects of CB 154 and perphenazine on adrenal function. *J. Endocrinol.,* 58:xxvii–xxviii.
20. Carlsson, A. (1975): Receptor mediated control of dopamine metabolism. In: *Pre- and Postsynaptic Receptors,* edited by E. Usdin and W. Bunney, pp. 49–65. Marcel Dekker, New York.
21. Caron, G. M., Beaulieu, M., Raymond, V., Gagne, B., Drouin, J., Lefkowitz, J., and Labrie, F. (1978): Dopaminergic receptors in the anterior pituitary gland. *J. Biol. Chem.,* 253:2244–2253.
22. Cerletti, A. (1959): Discussion contribution. *Neuropsychopharmacology,* 1:117–123.
23. Clark, B. J., and Menninger, K. (1980): Peripheral dopamine receptors. *Circ. Res. (Suppl. I)* 46 *(in press).*
24. Clark, B. J., Scholtysik, G., and Flückiger, E. (1978): Cardiovascular actions of bromocriptine. *Acta Endocrinol., (Kbh.),* 88(Suppl. 216):75–81.
25. Clark, J. H., and McCormack, Sh. (1977): Clomid or nafoxidine administered to neonatal rats causes reproductive tract abnormalities. *Science,* 197:164–165.
26. Colby, H. D. (1978): Effects of prolactin administration on adrenocorticol steroid metabolism in hypophysectomized female rats. *The Endocrine Society 60th Annual Meeting,* Abstract 290.
27. Corrodi, H., Farnebo, L. O., Fuxe, K., and Hamberger, B. (1975): Effect of ergot drugs on central 5-hydroxytryptamine neurons: Evidence for 5-hydroxytryptamine release or 5-hydroxytrytamine receptor stimulation. *Eur. J. Pharmacol.,* 30:172–181.

28. Corrodi, H., Fuxe, K., Hökfelt, T., Lidbrink, P., and Ungerstedt (1973): Effect of ergot drugs on central catecholamine neurons: Evidence for a stimulation of central dopamine neurons. *J. Pharm. Pharmacol.,* 25:409–411.
29. Costall, B., and Naylor, J. R. (1976): Apomorphine as an antagonist of the dopamine response from the nucleus accumbens. *J. Pharm. Pharmacol.,* 28:592–595.
30. Creese, I., Schneider, R., and Snyder, S. H. (1977): ^{3}H-spiroperidol labels dopamine receptors in pituitary and brain. *Eur. J. Pharmacol.,* 46:377–381.
31. Cronin, M. J., and Weiner, R. I., (1979): [^{3}H]Spiroperidol (spiperone) binding to a putative dopamine receptor in sheep and steer pituitary and stalk median eminence. *Endocrinology,* 104:307–312.
32. Davies, C., Jacobi, J., Lloyd, H. M., and Meares, J. D. (1974): DNA synthesis and the secretion of prolactin and growth hormone by the pituitary gland of the male rat: Effects of diethylstilbestrol and 2-bromo-α-ergocryptine methanesulphonate. *J. Endocrinol.,* 61:411–417.
33. De Camilli, P., Macconi, D., and Spada, A. (1979): Dopamine inhibits adenylate cyclase in human prolactin-secreting pituitary adenomas. *Nature,* 278:252–254.
34. Di Chiara, G., Porceddu, M. L., Vargiu, L., and Gessa, G. L. (1978): Stimulation of 'regulatory' dopamine receptors by bromocriptine (CB 154). *Pharmacology,* 16(Suppl. 1):135–142.
35. Eble, J. N. (1964): A proposed mechanism for the depressor effect of dopamine in the anaesthetised dog. *J. Pharmacol. Exp. Ther.,* 145:64–70.
36. Eckert, H., Kiechel, J. R., Rosenthaler, J., Schmidt, R., and Schreier, E. (1978): Biopharmaceutical aspects. In: *Ergot Alkaloids and Related Compounds. Handbook of Experimental Pharmacology, Vol. 49,* edited by B. Berde and H. O. Schild, pp. 719–803. Springer Verlag, Heidelberg.
37. Eikenburg, D. C., Ravitz, A. J., Gudelsky, G. A., and Moore, K. E. (1977): Effects of estrogen on prolactin and tuberoinfundibular dopaminergic neurons. *J. Neural Transm.,* 40:235–244.
38. Flückiger, E. (1972): Drugs and the control of prolactin secretion. Tenovus Workshop. In: *Prolactin and Carcinogenesis,* edited by A. R. Boyns and K. Griffiths, pp. 162–171. Alpha Omega Alpha Publishing, Cardiff, U.K.
39. Flückiger, E. (1976): The pharmacology of bromocriptine. In: *Pharmacological and Clinical Aspects of Bromocriptine (Parlodel),* edited by R. I. S. Bayliss, P. Turner, and W. P. Maclay, pp. 12–26. MCS Consultants, Tunbridge Wells, Kent, U.K.
40. Flückiger, E. (1978): Lactation inhibition by ergot drugs. In: *Physiology of Mammary Glands,* edited by A. Yokoyama, H. Mizuno, and H. Nagasawa, pp. 71–82. Japan Scientific Societies Press, Tokyo, and University Park Press, Baltimore.
41. Flückiger, E. (1978): Ergot alkaloids and the modulation of hypothalamic function. In: *Pharmacology of the Hypothalamus,* edited by B. Cox, I. D. Morris, and A. H. Weston, pp. 137–160. Macmillan, London.

42. Flückiger, E. (1980): Ergot and endocrine functions. In: *Ergot Alkaloids in Neurologic, Neuropsychiatric and Endocrine Disorders,* edited by M. Goldstein. Raven Press, New York *(in press).*
43. Flückiger, E., and del Pozo, E. (1978): Influence on the endocrine system. In: *Ergot Alkaloids and Related Compounds. Handbook of Experimental Pharmacology, Vol. 49,* edited by B. Berde and H. O. Schild, pp. 615–690. Springer Verlag, Heidelberg.
44. Flückiger, E., and Kovacs, E. (1974): Inhibition by 2-Br-α-ergokryptine-mesylate (CB 154) of suckling-induced pituitary prolactin depletion in lactating rats. *Experientia,* 30:1173.
45. Flückiger, E., Lutterbeck, P. M., Wagner, H. R., and Billeter, E. (1972): Antagonism of 2-Br-α-ergokryptine-methanesulphonate (CB 154) to certain endocrine actions of centrally active drugs. *Experientia,* 28:924–925.
46. Flückiger, E., Markó, M., Doepfner, W., and Niederer, W. (1976): Effects of ergot alkaloids on the hypothalamic-pituitary axis. *Postgrad. Med. J.,* 52(Suppl. 1):57–61.
47. Flückiger, E., and Vigouret, J. M. (1979): Drugs, dopamine and pituitary secretion. In: *Proceedings of the VIth International Symposium on Medicinal Chemistry,* edited by M. A. Simkins. Cotswold Press, Oxford.
48. Flückiger, E., Vigouret, J. M., and Wagner, H. R. (1978): Ergot compounds and prolactin secretion. In: *Progress in Prolactin Physiology and Pathology,* edited by C. Robyn and M. Harter, pp. 383–396. Elsevier/North-Holland Biomedical Press, Amsterdam.
49. Flückiger, E., and Wagner, H. (1968): 2-Br-α-Ergokryptin: Beeinflussung von Fertilität und Laktation bei der Ratte. *Experientia,* 24:1130–1131.
50. Friis, M. L., Grøn, U., Larsen, N. E., Pakkenberg, H., and Hvidberg, E. F. (1979): Pharmacokinetics of bromocriptine during continuous oral treatment of Parkinson's disease. *Eur. J. Clin. Pharmacol.,* 15:275–280.
51. Fuxe, K., Eneroth, P., Gustafsson, J. A., Löfström, A., and Skeet, P. (1977): Dopamine in the nucleus accumbens: Preferential increase of DA turnover by rat prolactin. *Brain Res.,* 122:177–182.
52. Fuxe, K., Fredholm, B. B., Ögren, S.-O., Agnati, L. F., Hökfelt, T., and Gustafsson, J.-A. (1978): Ergot drugs and central monoaminergic mechanisms: A histochemical, biochemical and behavioral analysis. *Fed. Proc.,* 37:2181–2191.
53. Fuxe, K., Löfström, A., Agnati, L. F., Everitt, B. J., Hökfelt, T., Jonsson, G., and Wiesel, F.-A. (1975): On the role of central catecholamine and 5-hydroxytryptamine neurons in neuroendocrine regulation. In: *Anatomical Neuroendocrinology,* edited by E. Stumpf and L. D. Grant, pp. 402–432. Karger, Basel.
54. Gautvik, K. M., Hoyt, R. F., Jr., and Tashjian, A. H. (1973): Effects of colchicine and 2-Br-α-ergokryptine-methanesulfonate (CB 154) on the release of prolactin and growth hormone by functional tumor cells in culture. *J. Cell. Physiol.,* 82:401–409.
55. Gibson, A., and Samini, M. (1978): Bromocriptine is a potent α-adrenoceptor antagonist in the perfused mesenteric blood vessels of the rat. *J. Pharm. Pharmacol.,* 30:314–315.

56. Goldstein, M., Lew, J. Y., Hata, F., and Lieberman, A. (1978): Binding interactions of ergot alkaloids with monoaminergic receptors in the brain. *Gerontology,* 24(Suppl. 1):76–85.
57. Goldstein, M., Lew, J. Y., Nakamura, S., Battista, A. F., Lieberman, A., and Fuxe, K. (1978): Dopaminephilic properties of ergot alkaloids. *Fed. Proc.,* 37:2202–2206.
58. Gorski, R. A., and Barraclough, C. A. (1963): Effects of low dosages of androgen on the differentiation of hypothalamic regulatory control of ovulation in the rat. *Endocrinology,* 73:210–216.
59. Grauwiler, J., and Griffith, R. W. (1974): Acute toxicity studies with 2-Br-α-ergokryptine mesylate (CB 154). *I.R.C.S. Med. Sci.,* 2:1516.
60. Griffith, R. W. (1974): Toxicity studies with 2-Br-α-ergocryptine mesylate (CB 154): Effects of prolonged oral administration in rats. *I.R.C.S. Med. Sci.,* 2:1661.
61. Griffith, R. W. (1976): Toxicity studies with 2-Bromo-α-ergokryptine (CB 154): Effects of prolonged oral administration in monkeys. *I.R.C.S. Med. Sci.,* 4:386.
62. Griffith, R. W. (1977): Bromocriptine and uterine neoplasia. *Br. Med. J.,* 2:1605.
63. Griffith, R. W., and Richardson, B. P. (1975): Toxicity studies with 2-bromo-α-ergokryptine (CB 154): Effects of prolonged oral administration in dogs. *I.R.C.S. Med. Sci.,* 3:298.
64. Grosvenor, C. E. (1956): Effect of ergotamine on milk-ejection in lactating rat. *Proc. Soc. Exp. Biol. (N.Y.),* 91:294–296.
65. Grosvenor, C. E., and Turner, Ch. W. (1956): Ergotamine, oxytocin and milk let-down in lactating rats. *Proc. Soc. Exp. Biol. (N.Y.),* 93:466–468.
66. Grosvenor, C. E., and Turner, Ch. W. (1957): Evidence for adrenergic and cholinergic components in milk let-down reflex in lactating rat. *Proc. Soc. Exp. Biol. (N.Y.),* 95:719–722.
67. Hafiez, A. A., Bartke, A., and Lloyd, C. W. (1972): The role of prolactin in the regulation of testis function: The synergistic effects of prolactin and luteinizing hormone on the incorporation of [1-^{14}C] acetate into testosterone and cholesterol by testes from hypophysectomized rats in vitro. *J. Endocrinol.,* 53:223–230.
68. Hamilton, J. M., Flaks, A., Saluja, P. G., and Maguire, S. (1975): Hormonally induced renal neoplasia in the male Syrian hamster and the inhibitory effect of 2-bromo-α-ergokryptine methanesulfonate. *J. Natl. Cancer Inst.,* 54:1385–1400.
69. Hart, I. C. (1973): Effect of 2-Br-α-ergokryptine on milk yield and the level of prolactin and growth hormone in the blood of the goat at milking. *J. Endocrinol.,* 57:179–180.
70. Häusler, A., Rohr, H. P., Marbach, P., and Flückiger, E. (1978): Changes in prolactin secretion in lactating rats assessed by correlative morphometric and biochemical methods. *J. Ultrastruct. Res.,* 64:74–84.
71. Hökfelt, T., and Fuxe, K. (1972): On the morphology and the neuroendocrine role of the hypothalamic catecholamine neurons. In: *Brain-Endocrine*

Interaction. Median Eminence: Structure and Function, edited by K. M. Knigge, D. E. Scott, and A. Weindl, pp. 181–223. Karger, Basel.
72. Horowski, R. (1978): Differences in the dopaminergic effects of the ergot derivatives bromocriptine, lisuride and *d*-LSD as compared to apomorphine. *Eur. J. Pharmacol.,* 51:157–166.
72*a*. Horowski, R. (1979): Hypothermic action of lisuride and differences to bromocriptine in the antagonistic effect of neuroleptics. *Naunyn Schmiedeberg's Arch. Pharmacol.,* 306:147–151.
73. Imbs, J. L., Schmit, M., and Schwartz, J.: Effets rénaux de la bromocriptine. *J. Pharmacol. (Paris), (in press).*
74. Ishibashi, M., and Yamaji, T. (1978): Effect of thyrotropin-releasing hormone and bromoergocriptine on growth hormone and prolactin secretion in perfused pituitary adenoma tissues of acromegaly. *J. Clin. Endocrinol. Metab.,* 47:1251–1256.
75. Johnson, A. M., Loew, D. M., and Vigouret, J. M. (1976): Stimulant properties of bromocriptine in comparison to apomorphine, *d*-amphetamine, and L-DOPA. *Br. J. Pharmacol.,* 56:59–68.
76. Kann, G., and Denamur, R. (1974): Possible role of prolactin during the oestrus cycle and gestation in the ewe. *J. Reprod. Fertil.,* 39:474–483.
77. Kann, G., and Martinet, J. (1975): Prolactin levels and duration of postpartum anoestrus in lactating ewes. *Nature,* 257:63–64.
78. Kebabian, J. W., and Calne, D. B. (1979): Multiple receptors for dopamine. *Nature,* 277:93–96.
79. Keller, H. H., and DaPrada, M. (1979): Central dopamine agonistic activity and microsomal biotransformation of lisuride, lergotrile and bromocriptine. *Life Sci.,* 24:1211–1222.
80. Kiechel, J.-R. (1980): Pharmacocinétique et métabolisme des dérivés de l'ergot. *J. Pharmacol. (Paris),* 10:533–565.
81. Kimura, H., Calabro, M. A., and MacLeod, R. M. (1976): Suppression of prolactin secretion and cAMP accumulation by dopamine in the pituitary. *Fed. Proc.,* 35:305.
82. Kordon, C. (1971): Blockade of ovulation in the immature rat by local microinjection of α-methyl-dopa into the arcuate region of the hypothalamus. *Neuroendocrinology,* 7:202–209.
83. Kovacs, E., and Flückiger, E. (1974): Influence of α-Br-α-ergokryptine-mesylate (CB 154) on the pituitary prolactin content of prooestrus rats. *Experientia,* 30:1172.
84. Labrie, F., Beaulieu, M., Caron, M. G., and Raymond, V. (1978): The adenohypophyseal dopamine receptor: Specificity and modulation of its activity by estradiol. In: *Progress in Prolactin Physiology and Pathology,* edited by C. Robyn and M. Harter, pp. 121–136. Elsevier/North-Holland Biomedical Press, Amsterdam and New York.
85. Lamberts, S. W. J., and MacLeod, R. M. (1979): The inability of bromocriptine to inhibit prolactin secretion by transplantable rat pituitary tumors: Observations on the mechanism and dynamics of the autofeedback regulation of prolactin secretion. *Endocrinology,* 104:65–70.

86. LeBlanc, H., Lachelin, G. C. L., Abu-Fadil, S., and Yen, S. S. C. (1977): The effect of dopamine infusion on insulin and glucagon secretion in man. *J. Clin. Endocrinol. Metab.,* 44:196–198.
87. Lew., J. Y., Hata, F., Ohashi, T., and Goldstein, M. (1977): The interaction of bromocriptine and lergotrile with dopamine and α-adrenergic receptors. *J. Neural Transm.,* 41:109–121.
88. Lichtensteiger, W., and Keller, P. J. (1974): Tubero-infundibular dopamine neurons and the secretion of luteinizing hormone and prolactin: Extrahypothalamic influences, interaction with cholinergic systems and the effect of urethane anesthesia. *Brain. Res.,* 74:279–303.
89. Liuzzi, A., Panerai, A. E., Chiodini, P. G., Secchi, C., Cocchi, D., Botalla, L., Silvestrini, F., and Müller, E. E. (1976): Neuroendocrine control of growth hormone secretion: Experimental and clinical studies. In: *Growth Hormone and Related Peptides,* edited by A. Pecile and E. E. Müller, pp. 236–251. Excerpta Medica, Amsterdam.
90. Lloyd, H. M., Jacoby, J. M., and Meares, J. D. (1978): DNA synthesis and depletion of prolactin in the pituitary gland of the male rat. *J. Endocrinol.,* 77:129–136.
91. Lloyd, H. M., Meares, J. D., and Jacobi, J. (1975): Effects of oestrogen and bromocriptine on *in vivo* secretion and mitosis in prolactin cells. *Nature,* 255:497–498.
92. Loew, D. M., van Deusen, E. B., and Meier-Ruge, W. (1978): Effects on the central neurons system. In: *Ergot Alkaloids and Related Compounds. Handbook of Experimental Pharmacology, Vol. 49,* edited by B. Berde and H. O. Schild, pp. 421–532. Springer Verlag, Heidelberg.
93. Loew, D. M., Vigouret, J. M., and Jaton, A. L. (1976): Neuropharmacological investigations with two ergot alkaloids, Hydergine and bromocriptine. *Postgrad. Med. J.,* 52(Suppl. 1):40–46.
94. Lorenzi, M., Karam, J. H., Tsalikian, E., Bohannon, N. V., Gerich, J. E., and Forsham, P. H. (1979): Dopamine during α- or β-adrenergic blockade in man. *J. Clin. Invest.,* 63:310–317.
95. Lutterbeck, P. M., Pryor, S., Varga, L., and Wenner, R. (1971): Treatment of non-puerperal galactorrhea with an ergot alkaloid. *Br. Med. J.,* 3:228–229.
96. MacLeod, R. M. (1976): Regulation of prolactin secretion. In: *Frontiers in Neuroendocrinology, Vol. IV,* edited by L. Martini and W. F. Ganong, pp. 169–194. Raven Press, New York.
97. Mahajan, K. K., Horrobin, D. F., and Robinson, C. J. (1975): Metbolic effects of 2-bromo-ergocryptine-methane-sulphonate (CB 154) in the rat. *J. Endocrinol.,* 64:587–588.
98. Mahajan, K. K., Manku, M. S., Davidson, H., James, M. F., Robinson, C. J., and Horrobin, D. F. (1976): Renal interaction of prolactin and bromocriptine. *J. Endocrinol.,* 68:14P.
99. Maj, J., Gancarczyk, L., and Rawlow, A. (1977): The influence of bromocriptine on serotonin neurons. *J. Neural Transm.,* 41:253–264.
100. Markó, M., and Flückiger, E. (1974): Inhibition of spontaneous and induced ovulation in rats by non-steroidal agents. *Experientia,* 30:1174–1176.

101. Markó, M., and Flückiger, E. (1976): Inhibition of ovulation in rats by antagonists to serotonin and by a new tricyclic compound. *Experientia,* 32:491–492.
102. Markó, M., and Flückiger, E. (1980): Role of serotonin in the regulation of ovulation: Evidence from pharmacological studies. *Neuroendocrinology,* 30:198–201.
103. Markstein, R., Herrling, P. L., Bürki, H. R., Asper, H., and Ruch, W. (1978): The effect of bromocripture on rat striatal adenylate cyclase and rat brain monoamine metabolism. *J. Neurochem.,* 31:1163–1172.
104. Markstein, R., Herrling, P., and Wagner, H. (1978): Bromocriptine mimics dopamine effects on the cyclic-AMP system of rat pituitary gland (Abstract). *Seventh International Congress of Pharmacology,* Paris. Pergamon Press Ltd.
105. Mashiter, K., Adams, E., Beard, M., and Holley, A. (1977): Bromocriptine inhibits prolactin and growth hormone release by human pituitary tumours in culture. *Lancet,* 2:197–199.
106. McCann, S. M. (1974): Regulation of secretion of follicle-stimulating hormone and luteinizing hormone. In: *Handbook of Physiology., Vol. IV,* edited by E. Knobil and W. H. Sawyer, pp. 489–518. American Physiological Society, Washington, D.C.
107. Meites, J., Huang, H. H., and Riegle, G. D. (1976): Relation of the hypothalamo-pituitary-gonadal system to decline of reproductive functions in aging female rats. In: *Hypothalamus and Endocrine Functions,* edited by F. Labrie, J. Meites, and G. Pelletier, pp. 3–20. Plenum Press, New York.
108. Milligan, J. V., and Kraicer, J. (1969): Calcium-45 uptake and potassium-induced release of ACTH from the adenohypophyses. *Physiologist,* 12:303.
109. Milligan, J. V., and Kraicer, J. (1970): Adenohypophyseal transmembrane potentials. Polarity reversal by elevated external potassium ion concentration. *Science,* 167:182–183.
110. Miyamoto, T., Battista, A., Goldstein, M., and Fuxe, K. (1974): Longlasting anti-tremor activity induced by 2-Br-α-ergokryptine in monkeys. *J. Pharm. Pharmacol.,* 26:452–454.
111. Montavani, P., Bartolini, A., and Pepeu, G. (1977): Interrelationship between dopaminergic and cholinergic systems in the cerebral cortex. Nonstriatal dopaminergic neurons. *Adv. Biochem. Psychopharmacol.,* 16:423–427.
112. Mowles, T. F., Burghardt, B., Burghardt, C., Charneki, A., and Sheppart, H. (1978): The dopamine receptor of the rat mammotroph in cell culture as a model for drug action. *Life Sci.,* 22:2103–2212.
113. Müller, E. E., Cocchi, D., Panerai, A. E., Gil-Ad, I., Locatelli, V., and Mantegazza, P. (1978): Pituitary hormones and ergot alkaloids. *Pharmacology,* 16(Suppl. 1):63–77.
114. Muller, G. G., and Kirk, R. W. (1969): *Small Animal Dermatology.* Saunders, Philadelphia.
115. Müller-Schweinitzer, E. (1976): Responsiveness of isolated canine cerebral and peripheral arteries to ergotamine. *Naunyn Schmiedeberg's Arch. Pharmacol.,* 295:41–44.

116. Müller-Schweinitzer, E., and Stürmer, E. (1972): Investigations on the mode of action of ergotamine in the isolated femoral vein of the dog. *Experientia,* 28:743.
117. Müller-Schweinitzer, E., and Weidmann, H. (1978): Basic pharmacological properties. In: *Ergot Alkaloids and Related Compounds. Handbook of Experimental Pharmacology, Vol. 49,* edited by B. Berde and H. O. Schild, pp. 87–232. Springer Verlag, Heidelberg.
118. Nagasawa, H., and Yanai, R. (1972): Promotion of pituitary prolactin release in rats by dibutyryl-adenosine 3′,5′-monophosphate. *J. Endocrinol.,* 55:215–217.
119. Nagasawa, H., Yanai, R., and Flückiger, E. (1973): Counteraction by 2-Br-α-ergokryptine of pituitary prolactin release promoted by dibutyryl-adenosine-3′,5′-monophosphate. In: *Human Prolactin,* edited by J. L. Pasteels and C. Robyn, pp. 313–315. Excerpta Medica, Amsterdam.
120. Nausieda, P. A., Weiner, W. J., Kanapa, D. J., and Klawans, H. L. (1978): Bromocriptine-induced behavioral hypersensitivity: Implications for the therapy of parkinsonism. *Neurology,* 28:1183–1188.
121. Niswender, G. D. (1974): Influence of 2-Br-α-ergocryptine on serum levels of prolactin and the oestrus cycle in sheep. *Endocrinology,* 94:612–615.
122. Olson, L., Fuxe, K., and Hökfelt, T. (1972): The effect of pituitary transplants on the tubero-infundibular dopamine neurons in various endocrine states. *Acta Endocrinol. (Kbh),* 71:233–244.
123. Pasteels, J. L., Danguy, A., Frérotte, M., and Ectors, F. (1971): Inhibition de la sécrétion de prolactine par l'ergocornine et la 2-Br-α-ergokryptine: Action directe sur l'hypophyse en culture. *Ann. Endocrinol. (Paris),* 32:188–192.
124. Pelletier, G., Lemay, A., Béraud, G., and Labrie, F. (1972): Ultrastructural changes accompanying the stimulatory effect of N^6-monobutyryl-adenosine-3′5′-monophosphate on the release of growth hormone (GH), prolactin (PRL) and adrenocorticotropic hormone (ACTH) in rat anterior pituitary gland *in vitro. Endocrinology,* 91:1355–1371.
125. Penny, R. J., and Thody, A. J. (1976): Preliminary studies on the control of α-melanocyte-stimulating hormone secretion in the rat. *J. Endocrinol.,* 69:2P–3P.
126. Penny, R. J., Tilders, F. J. H., and Thody, A. J. (1979): The role of the dopaminergic tubero-hypophyseal neurones in the maintenance of 'basal' melanocyte-stimulating hormone levels in the rat. *J. Endocrinol.,* 80:58P–59P.
127. Pepeu, G., and Mantovani, P. (1978): Effect of bromocriptine on acetylcholine output from the cerebral cortex. *Pharmacology,* 16(Suppl. 1):204–206.
128. Pijnenburg, A. J. J., Honig, W. M. M., Stuyker Boudier, J. A. J., Cools, A. R., Van der Heyden, J. A. M., and van Rossum, J. M. (1976): Further investigations on the effects of ergometrine and other ergot derivatives following injection into the nucleus accumbens of the rat. *Arch. Int. Pharmacodyn.,* 222:103–115.
129. Piva, F., Gagliano, P., Motta, M., and Martini, L. (1973): Adrenal progesterone factors controlling its secretion. *Endocrinology,* 93:1178–1184.

130. Portaleone, P. (1978): Bromocriptine and Hydergine: A comparison on striatal or hypothalamic adenylate cyclase activity. *Pharmacology,* 16(Suppl. 1):207–209.
131. Price, P., Debono, A., Parkes, J. D., Marsden, C. D., and Rosenthaler, J. (1978): Plasma bromocriptine levels, clinical and growth hormone responses in parkinsonism. *Br. J. Clin. Pharmacol.,* 6:303–309.
132. Puech, A. J., Simon, P., Chermat, R., and Boissier, J. R. (1977): Bromocriptine and methylergometrine: Pharmacological approach of the mechanism of their central effects. *Pharmacol. Res. Commun.,* 9:299–306.
133. Rand, M. J., Story, D. F., and McCulloch, M. W. (1975): Inhibitory feedback modulation of adrenergic transmission. *Clin. Exp. Pharmacol. Physiol.,* 2 Suppl.:21–26.
134. Rennels, F. G., and Callahan, W. P. (1959): The hormonal basis for pubertal maturation of the hair in the albino rat. *Anat. Rec.,* 135:21–27.
135. Richardson, B. P. (1973): Evidence for a physiological role of prolactin in osmoregulation in the rat. *Br. J. Pharmacol.,* 47:623P.
136. Rodway, R. G., and Kuhn, N. J. (1975): Luteal 20α-hydroxy steroid dehydrogenase and the formation of ^{4}-3-oxosteroids in the rat after weaning or treatment with 2-Bromo-α-ergocryptine during lactation. *Biochem. J.,* 152:445.
137. Rothlin, E., Cerletti, A., Konzett, H., Schalch, W. R., and Täschler, M. (1959): Zentrale vegetative LSD-Effekte. *Experientia,* 12:154–155.
138. Saameli, K. (1978): Effects on the uterus. In: *Ergot Alkaloids and Related Compounds. Handbook of Experimental Pharmacology, Vol. 49,* edited by B. Berde and H. O. Schild, pp. 233–319. Springer Verlag, Heidelberg.
139. Schams, D. (1972): Prolactin release effects of TRH in the bovine and their depression by a prolactin inhibitor. *Horm. Metab. Res.,* 4:405.
140. Schmidt, M. J., and Hill, L. E. (1977): Effects of ergots on adenylate cyclase activity in the corpus striatum and pituitary. *Life Sci.,* 20:789–798.
141. Schneider, H. R., Stadler, P. A., Stütz, P., and Troxler, F. (1977): Synthese und Eigenschaften von Bromocriptin. *Experientia,* 33:1412–1413.
142. Scholtysik, G. (1976): Dopaminergic inhibition of the function of postganglionic adrenergic heart nerves in cats. *Naunyn Schmiedeberg's Arch. Pharmacol.,* 293(Suppl.):R2.
143. Scholtysik, G. (1978): Dopamine receptor mediated inhibition by bromocriptine of accelerator nerve stimulation effects in the pithed cat. *Br. J. Pharmacol.,* 62:379P.
144. Schorderet, M. (1978): Dopamine-mimetic activity of ergot derivatives, as measured by the production of cyclic-AMP in isolated retinae of the rabbit. *Gerontology,* 24(Suppl. 1):86–93.
145. Schran, H. F., Suryakant, I. B., Schwarz, H. J., and Loeffler, L. J. (1979): Development and application of a specific radioimmunoassay for the dopamine receptor agonist bromocriptine. *J. Clin. Chem.,* 25:1928–1933.
146. Schran, H. F., Suryakant, I. B., Schwarz, H. J., and Thorner, M. O.: The pharmacokinetics of bromocriptine in man. In: *Ergot Alkaloids in*

Neurologic, Neuropsychiatric and Endocrine Disorders, edited by M. Goldstein. Raven Press, New York *(in press).*
147. Schriefers, H., Keck, E., Klein, S., and Schröder, E. (1975): Die Funktion der Hypophyse und des Hypophysenhormons Prolaktin für die Aufrechterhaltung der Sexualspezifität des Stoffwechsels von Testosteron und 5-α-Dihydrotestosteron in Rattenleberschnitten. *Hoppe Seyler's Z. Physiol. Chem.,* 356:1535–1543.
148. Schriefers, H., and Wagner, W. (1976): Cholesterol 7α-hydroxylase activity of the rat liver after hypophysectomy and administration of hypophyseal hormones. *Experientia,* 32:18–19.
149. Seybold, V. S., Miller, J. W., and Lewis, P. R. (1978): Investigation of a dopaminergic mechanism for regulating oxytocin release. *J. Pharm. Exp. Ther.,* 207:605–610.
150. Shelesnyak, M. C. (1954): Ergotoxine inhibition of deciduoma formation and its reversal by progesterone. *Am. J. Physiol.,* 179:301–304.
151. Shelesnyak, M. C. (1975): Comments. In: *Pioneers in Neuroendocrinology,* edited by J. Meites, B. T. Donovan, and S. M. McCann, pp. 267–278. Plenum Press, New York.
152. Silbergeld, E. K., Adler, H., Kennedy, S., and Calne, D. B. (1977): The role of presynaptic function and hepatic drug metabolism in the hypothermic actions of two novel dopaminergic agonists. *J. Pharm. Pharmacol.,* 29:632–635.
153. Sinha, Y. N., Selby, F. W., and Vanderlaan, W. P. (1974): Effects of ergot drugs on prolactin and growth hormone secretion, and on mammary nucleic acid content in C3H/Bi mice. *J. Natl. Cancer Inst.,* 52:189–191.
154. Smith, V. G., Beck, T. W., Convey, E. M., and Tucker, H. A. (1974): Bovine serum prolactin, growth hormone, cortisol and milk yield after ergocryptine. *Neuroendocrinology,* 15:172–181.
155. Smythe, G. A., Brandstater, J. F., Compton, P. J., and Lazarus, L. (1977): *In vivo* and *in vitro* inhibition of monoamine oxidase activity in the rat by 2-bromo-α-ergocryptine. In: *Twentieth Annual Meeting, The Endocrine Society of Australia,* Abstract No. 12. P. E. Harding, Adelaide.
156. Snider, S. R., Hutt, C., Stein, B., and Fahn, S. (1975): Increase in brain serotonin produced by bromocriptine. *Neurosci. Lett.,* 1:237.
157. Stürmer, E., and Flückiger, E. (1974): *In vivo* smooth muscle stimulating activity of 2-Br-α-ergokryptine-mesylate (CB 154) as compared with that of ergotamine. *IRCS, Med. Sci.,* 2:1591.
158. Tashjian, A. H., and Hoyt, R. F. (1972): Transient control of organ specific functions in pituitary cells in culture. In: *Molecular Genetics and Developmental Biology,* edited by M. Sussman, pp. 353–387. Prentice Hall, Englewood Cliffs.
159. Tashjian, A. H., Lomedico, M. E., and Maina, D. (1978): Role of calcium in the thyrotropin-releasing hormone-stimulated release of prolactin from pituitary cells in culture. *Biochem. Biophys. Res. Commun.,* 81:798–806.
160. Titeler, M., Weinreich, P., Sinclair, D., and Seeman, P. (1978): Multiple receptors for brain dopamine. *Proc. Natl. Acad. Sci. U.S.A.,* 75:1153–1156.

161. Trabucchi, M., Hofmann, M., Montefusco, O., and Spano, P. F. (1978): Ergot alkaloids and cyclic nucleotides in the CNS. *Pharmacology,* 16 (Suppl. 1):150–155.
162. Trabucchi, M., Spano, P. F., Tonon, G. C., and Fratolla, L. (1976): Effects of bromocriptine on central dopaminergic receptors. *Life Sci.,* 19:225–232.
163. Ungerstedt, U. (1971): Postsynaptic supersensitivity after 6-hydroxydopamine induced degeneration of the nigro-neostriatal dopamine system. *Acta Physiol. Scand.,* Suppl. 367:69–73.
164. Varga, L., Lutterbeck, P. M., Pryor, J. S., Wenner, R., and Erb, H. (1972): Suppression of puerperal lactation with an ergot alkaloid: A double-blind study. *Br. Med. J.,* 2:743–744.
165. Vigouret, J. M., Bürki, H. R., Jaton, A. L., Züger, P. E., and Loew, D. M. (1978): Neurochemical and neuropharmacological investigations with four ergot derivatives: Bromocriptine, dihydroergotoxine, CF 25-397 and CM 29–712. *Pharmacology,* 16(Suppl. 1):156–173.
166. Vigouret, J. M., Jaton, A. L., and Loew D. M. (1979): Increased sensitivity after repeated administration of ergot derivatives in rat. *Experientia,* 37:41.
167. Weiner, W. J., Nausieda, P. A., and Klawans, H. L. (1978): The effect of levodopa, lergotrile, and bromocriptine on brain iron, manganese, and copper. *Neurology,* 28:734–737.
168. West, B., and Dannies, P. S. (1979): Antipsychotic drugs inhibit prolactin release from rat anterior pituitary cells in culture by a mechanism not involving the dopamine receptor. *Endocrinology,* 104:877–880.
169. Witorsch, R. J., and Edwards, J. T. (1976): Comparison of effects of prolactin and growth hormone on adrenal 5α-reductase in hypophysectomized rats. *Proc. Soc. Exp. Biol. Med.,* 151:689–693.
170. Witorsch, R. J., and Kitay, J. I. (1972): Pituitary hormones affecting adrenal 5α-reductase activity: ACTH, growth hormone and prolactin. *Endocrinology,* 91:764–769.
171. Yanai, R., and Nagasawa, H. (1970*a*): Suppression of mammary hyperplastic nodule formation and pituitary prolactin secretion in mice induced by ergocornine and 2-Br-α-ergocryptine. *J. Natl. Cancer Inst.,* 45:1105–1112.
172. Yanai, R., and Nagasawa, H. (1970*b*): Effects of ergocornine and 2-Br-α-ergocryptine (CB 154) on the formation of mammary hyperplastic alveolar nodules and the pituitary prolactin levels in mice. *Experientia,* 26:649–650.
173. Yanai, R., and Nagasawa, H. (1974): Effect of 2-Br-α-ergocryptine on pituitary synthesis and release of prolactin and growth hormone in rats. *Horm. Res.,* 5:1–5.
174. Yeh, B. J., McNay, J. L., and Goldberg, L. I. (1969): Attenuation of dopamine renal and mesenteric vasodilation by haloperidol: Evidence for a specific receptor. *J. Pharmacol. Exp. Ther.,* 168:303–309.
175. Yeo, T., Thorner, M. O., Jones, A., Lowry, P. J., and Besser, G. M. (1979): The effects of dopamine, bromocriptine, lergotrile and metoclo-

pramide on prolactin release from continuously perfused columns of isolated rat pituitary cells. *Clin. Endocrinol.,* 10:123–130.

176. Zeilmaker, G. H., and Carlsen, R. A. (1962): Experimental studies on the effect of ergocornine methanesulfonate on the luteotrophic function of the rat pituitary gland. *Acta Endocrinol. (Kbh.),* 41:321.
177. Ziegler, M. G., Lake, C. R., Williams, A. C., Teychenne, P. F., Shoulson, I., and Steinsland, O. (1979): Bromocriptine inhibits norepinephrine release. *Clin. Pharmacol. Ther.,* 25:137–142.
178. Zor, U., Kaneko, T., Schneider, H. P. G., McCann, S. M., and Field, J. B. (1970): Further studies of stimulation of anterior pituitary cyclic adenosine-3′,5′-monophosphate formation by hypothalamic extracts and prostaglandins. *J. Biol. Chem.,* 245:2883–2888.

3

Bromocriptine Therapy for Hyperprolactinemia and Suppression of Puerperal Lactation

I. INTRODUCTION TO DISORDERS OF PROLACTIN SECRETION

Human prolactin is secreted by the anterior pituitary and has a molecular weight of 23,500, which is similar to that of growth hormone (108). Prolactin was identified as separate and distinct from growth hormone in 1970 (45,46,51), and 1 year later it was isolated and purified (67). The isolation was difficult, first because of the similarity of the molecular weights of prolactin and growth hormone; second, the pituitary content of prolactin is only one-tenth that of growth hormone; and third, the lactogenic potency of growth hormone is equivalent to that of prolactin in bioassays used to follow the purification process. However, the purification of small quantities of human prolactin by Friesen and colleagues made possible the generation of antibodies and thus the development of simple, sensitive, specific, and reliable radioimmunoassays (71).

In 1977 Shome and Parlow (108) published the amino acid sequence of human prolactin. It has only 15% homology of structure with human growth hormone, but there is 80% homology with prolactins from other species.

Initially through the use of sensitive bioassays, and later through radioimmunoassays, the knowledge of the physiology of human prolactin advanced quickly, and it became clear that disorders of prolactin secretion are not rare; in fact, they are probably the most common disorders of hypothalamic/pituitary function (50,52,113). Coincidentally, bromocriptine, a drug that had been developed specifically to inhibit prolactin secretion (43), was introduced into clinical research. The story of prolactin and bromocriptine are inextricably interwoven.

II. CONTROL OF PROLACTIN SECRETION

Secretion of anterior pituitary hormones is regulated by the hypothalamus and by feedback effects of the secretory products from their target glands (Fig. 1). The hypothalamus regulates

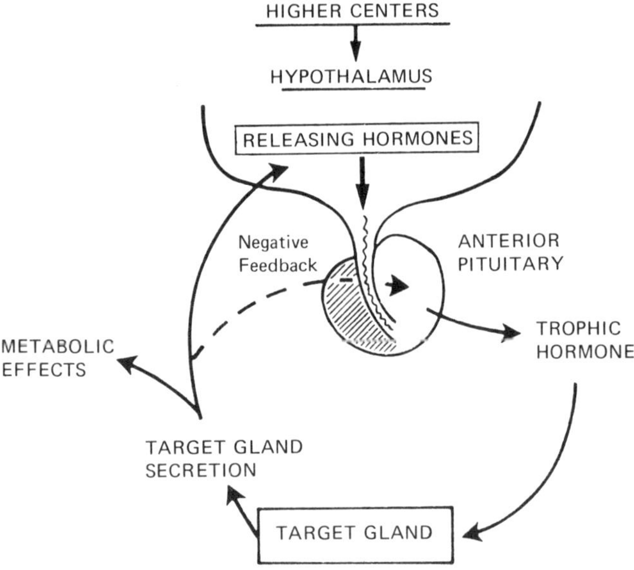

FIG. 1. Diagrammatic representation of the relationships between the hypothalamic regulatory hormones and their actions on the pituitary. Secretion, or inhibition of tonic secretion, of specific trophic hormones occurs, which in turn influences secretion of the target organ hormones. These target hormones may modify pituitary hormone secretion by the feedback control mechanism either at the hypothalamic level or by interfering with the action of the regulatory hormones on the pituitary cells. (Reproduced with permission from Hall et al., ref. 68a.)

anterior pituitary hormone secretion by synthesizing hypothalamic regulatory hormones, which are released at the median eminence into the capillaries of the hypothalamo-hypophyseal portal capillary system. In this way, these factors are transported to the cells of the anterior pituitary, where they exert their specific effects on specific cells. Thus, for example, the gonadotropin releasing hormone only stimulates the pituitary gonadotrophs to secrete FSH and LH. This system links the central nervous and endocrine systems and is a beautiful example of the great sophistication and yet simplicity of the evolution of higher organisms. Apart from allowing for very fine homeostatic control, the hypothalamus-pituitary-target organ system acts as a cascade amplifier; very small quantities of hypothalamic regulatory hormones are synthesized and released to stimulate larger quantities of anterior pituitary hormones, which in turn stimulate the production and release of even larger quanitities of target gland secretions. Unlike other pituitary hormones, such as thyrotropin and corticotropin, prolactin has no obvious peripheral target gland and thus the factors that control feedback in prolactin secretion are unclear. It is known that prolactin feeds back on itself (short-loop feedback) and that two hypothalamic factors, a prolactin releasing factor (PRF), and a prolactin release inhibiting factor(s) (PIF), regulate prolactin release. Prolactin is unique among the anterior pituitary hormones in being under tonic hypothalamic *inhibition.* Thus, if there is disruption of the connection between the pituitary and the hypothalamus—for example, by stalk section—secretion of all the anterior pituitary hormones will become deficient, with the exception of prolactin, which will be secreted in excess (41,112,113).

Prolactin releasing factor. This substance has yet to be isolated. Thyrotropin-releasing hormone (TRH) is a potent releasor of prolactin, but is thought to be physiologically unimportant, since the release of prolactin, either during sleep or after suckling, occurs independently of thyrotropin (58). Furthermore, PRF activity can be identified in hypothalamic extracts that are devoid of TRH (54,81,124).

Prolactin release inhibiting factor. The isolation of a peptide PIF has not been achieved. There is now abundant evidence that at least one, and probably the most important, physiological PIF is the catecholamine dopamine (86,113). It was clear from early studies that dopamine was implicated in the inhibition of prolactin release. Administration of dopamine led to an increase in PIF activity in the hypothalamus. Dopamine, when added *in vitro* to rat hemipituitaries, inhibited prolactin release (87). Furthermore, Schally and colleagues, in their attempts at isolating a peptide PIF, found their most potent fraction to be devoid of peptide, containing only the catecholamines norepinephrine and dopamine (104). Dopamine, in concentrations that produce inhibition of prolactin release *in vitro,* is detectable in portal blood from the rat (60), and dopamine receptors are present on lactotroph cells in the pituitary (13,14,25).

Complicating the subject are the following reports: (a) PIF activity occurs in hypothalamic extracts, and its biological effect cannot be completely blocked by dopamine receptor blocking drugs (37); (b) adsorption of dopamine in hypothalamic extracts does not neutralize all PIF activity (38); and (c) gamma aminobutyric acid in very high concentration (10^{-5} M) can partially inhibit prolactin release *in vitro* (84,105).

Irrespective of the final outcome of the controversy, dopamine is clearly an important, physiologically active PIF, and from a clinical viewpoint may be considered the most important. This is schematically illustrated in Fig. 2; the hypothalamus tonically inhibits prolactin release by secreting dopamine directly at the median eminence into the portal capillaries to inhibit prolactin release from the lactotroph cells in the adenohypophysis.

The mechanism by which dopamine inhibits prolactin release from these cells is still not clear. However, dopamine effects are probably independent of cyclic AMP *(see page 32).* Recently, Douglas and associates showed electrical activity at membranes of fish and mammalian anterior pituitary cells; these cells are presumably lactotrophs (111). The action potentials (spikes) of

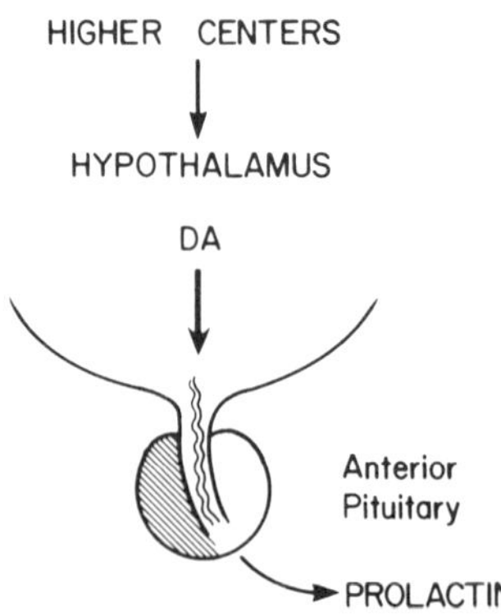

FIG. 2. Diagrammatic representation of tonic hypothalamic inhibition of prolactin secretion by dopamine.

these cells have been proposed to act as the excitatory drive for secretory activity (33,111). Dopamine has been shown to inhibit the frequency of these spikes, although the mechanism by which it achieves this inhibition is not clear (33). As in neuronal tissue and other endocrine cells, prolactin secretion is dependent on exocytosis, which requires calcium ions. Spiking may also require calcium ions. Recently, we investigated these phenomena using D-600, a drug that blocks regenerative calcium spikes but may not block calcium necessary for exocytosis (68,121). It was possible to demonstrate that prolactin release is blocked by this compound. We have proposed that dopamine acts by interfering with plasma membrane calcium permeability, either by blocking calcium-dependent spikes or by directly interfering with the exocytotic process (121).

The secretory patterns of prolactin secretion have been extensively studied and reviewed (112,113). Prolactin levels rise during the early hours of sleep and, like growth hormone and ACTH, during physical or psychological stress. During pregnancy, in response to rising estradiol levels, prolactin levels increase to approximately 500 ng/ml (normal for nonpregnant woman is less than 20 ng/ml) in the third trimester. Under the influence of prolactin, estrogen, and progesterone, the breast is prepared for lactation, but milk does not come into the breast until 2 to 3 days after delivery, when the endogenous gonadal steroid levels fall. In the postpartum woman, suckling leads to a marked rise in prolactin levels over 30 min (94). The levels then fall progressively. In women in the western world, the basal level and the response to suckling decline progressively as the interval from delivery increases (94). In contrast, in more primitive cultures, where breast feeding is the sole source of nutrition for the baby, prolactin levels remain elevated for longer. Furthermore, the response to suckling in these women does not diminish to the same degree as in their western counterparts; this difference may be due to more frequent and vigorous suckling. At the end of 1 year, serum prolactin levels remain elevated, providing a natural form of contraception not enjoyed by western women (30,52,109).

III. CAUSES OF HYPERPROLACTINEMIA

From the discussion of the control of prolactin secretion, the causes of hyperprolactinemia are readily comprehensible. Either too little dopamine is synthesized, too little is delivered to the lactotroph cells, or the lactotroph cells are insensitive to its effect, e.g., after being exposed to a dopamine receptor blocking drug (Table 1).

The ingestion of drugs that either deplete central dopamine stores or block dopamine receptors, and of estrogens, which act directly at the pituitary, has often been reported as the most common cause of hyperprolactinemia in clinical practice. Today, small tumors of the pituitary—microadenomata—are probably the most common cause of hyperprolactinemia. There are many unresolved questions about microadenomata. Nothing is known about their development. They appear to be rare in men, or per-

TABLE 1. *Causes of hyperprolactinemia*

Hypothalamic dopamine deficiency
disease of hypothalamus
tumor
a–v malformation
infiltration
drugs
α methyl dopa
reserpine
Interference with dopamine delivery to pituitary
stalk section
microadenoma
macroadenoma
Lactotroph insensitivity to dopamine
microadenoma or macroadenoma
drugs
phenothiazines
butyrophenones
Stimulation of lactotroph cells
estrogens
TRH (hypothyroidism)

haps go undiagnosed; hyperprolactinemia in men is almost always associated with large pituitary tumors (macroadenomata). Do these tumors lead to hyperprolactinemia because they lose their sensitivity to dopamine, or is the dopamine not released at the median eminence or not transported to the cells as a result of distorted anatomy within the tumor? Dopamine receptors have been demonstrated on human lactotroph cells from adenomata, and appear to be normal (25a). Furthermore, prolactin levels are lowered, usually to normal, by bromocriptine, which acts on dopamine receptors irrespective of whether or not an obvious pituitary tumor is present (6,28,114,115).

Since it is now becoming clear that hyperprolactinemia is an extremely common disease, the question has been posed by several groups as to the cause of the current "epidemic" (99). One factor that has been suggested as possibly being etiologically important is the widespread use of estrogen-containing oral contraceptives (107). Two published studies investigated this theory and could not find evidence to support it (24,74). Before any factor can be invoked it must be shown that the incidence is increasing. Since the technology to diagnose this condition has been available for only 6 to 9 years, it is obviously impossible to prove any causative factor, because no change in incidence has been shown. Clearly, in patients with this disorder, it had been present for years but remained undiagnosed. This point is well illustrated when patients treated with exogenous gonadotropins are reinvestigated and many are found to be hyperprolactinemic. If these patients are treated with bromocriptine, their gonadal function and fertility are restored to normal.

IV. CLINICAL FEATURES OF HYPERPROLACTINEMIA

Patients with hyperprolactinemia may present with symptoms related to their hormonal disturbance, or more rarely, with local symptoms referable to a pituitary tumor—headaches or visual field defects. Hyperprolactinemia, as mentioned previously, is diagnosed much less frequently in men than in women. In men, the clinical presentation is generally related either to problems due to local extension of the pituitary tumor or to secondary deficiencies of thyroid, cortisol, or testosterone; relative or absolute impotence is generally present and may be related either to the low testosterone levels or to a direct effect of hyperprolactinemia. The mechanisms involved are poorly understood.

Galactorrhea, either spontaneous or found only on examination by the physician, occurs in approximately 30% of hyperprolactinemic men and women (49,119). In some series, including our own, galactorrhea was found in over 80% of patients (69,114). Furthermore, many women with galactorrhea have normal prolactin levels; therefore, galactorrhea is a poor marker of hyperprolactinemia.

The menstrual patterns in women with hyperprolactinemia are variable, ranging from regular cycles, with or without an abnormal luteal phase, to polymenorrhea, oligomenorrhea, and most commonly, amenorrhea (114). Many amenorrheic patients complain of loss of libido, dyspareunia, depression, and personality changes. As patients are treated their symptoms recede.

There is a small group of hyperprolactinemic women who have symptoms and signs suggestive of the polycystic ovary syndrome. For the most part these patients have only mild hirsutism. This symptom complex is probably related to the effects of prolactin on the adrenal cortex, which are discussed below.

V. MECHANISMS OF HYPOGONADISM INDUCED BY HYPERPROLACTINEMIA

In the presence of hyperprolactinemia, testosterone levels in men are depressed, and this abnormality is accompanied by, but does not necessarily cause, loss of libido and of potency (the ability to have an erection) (15,48,92,114,119). In women, ovulation usually ceases and varying degrees of estrogen deficiency develop in association with vaginal dryness and dyspareunia (8,49).

At present, four hypotheses have been put forward to account for the suppression of gonadal function in hyperprolactinemia: (a) suppression of gonadotropin secretion; (b) altered positive feedback of estrogen on LH secretion in women; (c) changes in adrenal androgen secretion; and (d) blockade of the effects of gonadotropins at the gonadal level. The four mechanisms are discussed in some detail below. However, it should be pointed out that the problem of hypogonadism may well result from some combination of abnormalities or from other as yet undefined alterations in the hypothalamic-pituitary-gonadal axis.

Suppression of gonadotropin secretion. Patients with hyperprolactinemia generally have LH and FSH levels in the normal range for men and in the normal follicular phase range for women (8,49,114). However, in men the serum testosterone levels are usually low and in women, serum estradiol levels may vary from low (i.e., compatible with the postmenopausal state) to those seen in the follicular phase of the menstrual cycle. Gonadotropin secretion is dependent on stimulation by the hypothalamic decapeptide gonadotropin releasing hormone (GnRH) and by feedback effects of gonadal steroids. In view of the decreased circulating levels of gonadal steroids in hyperprolactinemia, some have argued that the gonadotropin levels are not normal but are actually low (73); it is not possible to determine whether the levels seen are appropriate or not.

Studies of women with hyperprolactinemia have shown normal or excessive gonadotropin responses to a supramaximal dose of GnRH compared to women in the follicular phase of the cycle (8,91,114).

Using a more sophisticated approach of either infusion of low doses of GnRH or, alternatively, repeated low dose bolus injections every 2 hr, Yen and colleagues delineated two pools of LH—a readily releasable pool (pool 1), and a storage pool (pool 2), similar to those proposed for insulin secretion (70,131). Using these techniques, they observed the following in normal women:

1. During the early follicular phase of the cycle, pools 1 and 2 were at a minimum (subsequent changes are described in comparison to the early follicular phase).

2. At the midfollicular phase of the cycle, there was a doubling of pool 2, with no change in pool 1.

3. In the late follicular phase a threefold increase in pool 1 and fivefold increase in pool 2 were observed.

4. On the day of the midcycle LH surge, there was a preferential ninefold increase in pool 1 and only a doubling of pool 2, as compared to the late follicular phase. At midcycle, the pattern of LH release during a 4-hr infusion suggested that release was greater than synthesis.

5. In the midluteal phase of the cycle, the first pool was very small, like that of the early follicular phase, and the second pool was similar to that of the late follicular phase.

On the basis of these observations, and of studies using infusions followed by bolus injections of submaximal doses of GnRH in normal women, Yen has proposed the following model to explain these phenomena (Fig. 3): (a) GnRH has a positive effect on synthesis, storage, and release of LH and on activation of transport from storage to releasable pools. (b) Estradiol is operative only in the presence of GnRH and may both stimulate synthesis and storage and impair release of LH (except possibly at midcycle).

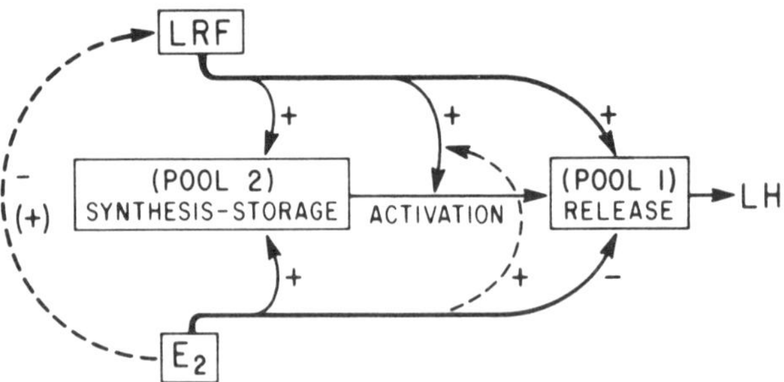

FIG. 3. Schematic representation of Yen's proposition of two pools of LH in gonadotrophs and the influence of the gonadotropin releasing hormone (GnRH) and estradiol (E_2) on them. Pool 1 = releasable pool; pool 2 = synthesis and storage pool of LH. (Reproduced with permission from Yen, ref. 134.)

The rise in the storage pool during follicular development is associated with increasing estradiol levels. At midcycle the increase in the releasable pool may be directly related to mounting stimulation by GnRH. This observed increase in effect of GnRH may be due either to actual increases in GnRH itself or to increased sensitivity of the gonadotroph to GnRH—the so-called self-priming effect. Either of these may be facilitated by estradiol.

The fall in the releasable pool during the midluteal phase of the cycle has been explained by decreasing amounts of GnRH reaching the pituitary during this phase of the cycle, but could as well be explained by decreased sensitivity to GnRH owing to the changing gonadal steroid environment.

Using a similar overall experimental design, Yen has shown that the pituitary LH sensitivity to GnRH and reserve are diminished in hyperprolactinemic patients compared to women in the follicular phase of the cycle (82). Although estrogen levels were low, basal levels of LH and FSH were similar to those seen in normal women in the follicular phase of the cycle. However, there was an increased release of FSH in response to GnRH as compared to normal women in the follicular phase of the cycle. This pattern of the alteration of LH to FSH ratio in favor of FSH could be explained by the reduction in estradiol levels, or more likely, by reduced GnRH; this is reminiscent of the secretory pattern of gonadotropins seen in early puberty. Furthermore, in patients with hyperprolactinemia, pulsatility of LH secretion is lost (8,9). Since the response of the gonadotroph to exogenous GnRH appears to be intact, it is necessary to propose altered GnRH release in these patients.

In the rat, the elevation of prolactin levels, either by injection or by transplantation of pituitary tissue under the renal capsule, leads to an increase in dopamine turnover in the hypothalamus (57). Anatomically, there is a close relationship between the dopaminergic and GnRH neurons in the lateral palazade zone of the hypothalamus. Based on that association and the fact that in hyperprolactinemic rats, pituitary LH content is reduced, Fuxe has suggested that dopamine inhibits GnRH release (57).

Although there are many *in vivo* and *in vitro* reports to suggest a stimulatory role for dopamine on GnRH release in the rat, there are no such data in man. Yen has produced convincing evidence of an inhibitory role for dopamine in normal women, the effect of dopamine infusions being most marked at day 14 of the menstrual cycle (76). In hyperprolactinemic women, it would follow that dopaminergic inhibition of GnRH would be maximal. In this situation, metoclopramide, a dopamine antagonist, has been shown to stimulate LH release, an effect not seen in normal women (98). Furthermore, as would be predicted from this model, Evans and colleagues (40) were unable to inhibit LH release with bromocriptine in hyperprolactinemic women, in contrast to the report of Lachelin and colleagues (83). The concept of inhibition of GnRH release by dopamine is attractive, since it could account for the loss of spiking of LH and the development of amenorrhea with inappropriately low LH levels, although pituitary reserve in response to pharmacologic doses of GnRH remains "normal."

Suppression of positive feedback by estrogen on LH secretion. In normal adult women, the administration of estrogen for several days leads initially to lowering of LH levels, followed by a surge of LH secretion after 48 to 72 hr. The same phenomenon can be demonstrated in other primates. Glass and associates have shown that in hyperprolactinemic women, negative feedback is intact but positive feedback is suppressed (62). It has been shown that positive feedback is restored when prolactin levels are lowered with bromocriptine therapy or by removal of the prolactin secreting tumor (42). This reduction in serum prolactin is followed by restoration of regular menstrual cycles.

Whether or not the absence of a positive feedback effect of estrogen in hyperprolactinemia represents a further abnormality of hypothalamic–pituitary function different from that described above for suppression of gonadotropin secretion remains to be seen. Positive feedback depends not only on intact gonadotroph function, but also on GnRH release. Thus, if GnRH release is impaired by feedback of prolactin, that in itself might account for the absence of positive feedback.

Prolactin and adrenal androgen secretion. In man, the role of prolactin in adrenocortical function is unclear. In lower vertebrates, prolactin has been shown to be important in the control of steroidogenesis in the maintenance of steroid precursor pools (1,93); it also has corticotropic effects (18). Adrenalectomy leads to increased prolactin secretion in rats (3), and hyperprolactinemic mice have hyperplastic adrenal glands (55).

In man, corticosteroids can partially inhibit prolactin secretion (21,80). Ovine prolactin was reported to restore responsiveness of the adrenal to ACTH in one woman (72), and a similar effect has been demonstrated *in vitro* with isolated rat adrenal cells (85).

The strongest data in favor of a role for prolactin in adrenal cortical function in man come from observations in hyperprolactinemic women. Forbes and colleagues (44) noted that 24-hr urinary 17 ketosteroid excretion was often increased in the galactorrhea/amenorrhea syndrome. This observation has been confirmed by others and these findings, together with clinical observations that patients with hyperprolactinemia may have clinical features suggestive of the polycystic ovary syndrome, have stimulated a reinvestigation of the role of prolactin in adrenal androgen secretion, using more specific assays (63,116). Several groups have noticed an increase in circulating dehydroepiandrosterone sulphate (DHEAS) levels in patients with hyperprolactinemia (16,-61,114,126). Desphande (32), studying the effects of ACTH and TRH (and thus prolactin) on adrenal cortical function, found that whereas ACTH raised both plasma pregnenolone and dehydroepiandrostenedione (DHEA), pregnenolone was preferentially affected. TRH increased only DHEA, suggesting a direct stimulation by TRH and/or prolactin on adrenal androgen production.

The several studies in hyperprolactinemic women that have shown elevated levels of DHEAS also show increased levels of DHEA. Similar observations have been made in men, in postmenopausal women with spontaneous hyperprolactinemia, in normal women in whom hyperprolactinemia has been induced with prolonged psychotropic drug administration, in women during the luteal phase, and in postmenopausal women (126). However,

Thorner and colleagues (119) were unable to alter circulating adrenal androgen levels in two normal men with hyperprolactinemia induced with metoclopramide for 1 month. In the woman with hyperprolactinemia, the levels of DHEAS and DHEA could be lowered either by removal of the prolactin secreting tumor or by lowering prolactin levels with bromocriptine (16,61).

Elevation of DHEAS and/or DHEA levels might result from either increased production or decreased metabolism. Although the former appears to be more likely, the latter has not been excluded. The increased urinary excretion of DHEA shown by Giusti and associates (61) in hyperprolactinemic women, and the increased 17 ketosteroid excretion reported previously, lend strong support to the increased production theory. If this is the case, the most likely source for these androgens is the adrenal gland; normally, the majority of DHEA and more than 90% of DHEAS come from the adrenal. Furthermore, elevated levels were seen in ovariectomized hyperprolactinemic women (126). Since Giusti and colleagues found elevated levels of only delta 5 androgens (androstendiol, DHEA and DHEAS) and not of delta 4 androgens (androstendione and testosterone), they have suggested that chronic hyperprolactinemia effects mainly the delta 5 pathway (61).

Blockade of gonadotropin effects at the gonadal level by prolactin. The prolactin concentration in human follicular fluid of the ovarian-Graafian follicle changes at different stages of the menstrual cycle. The lowest levels were observed just prior to ovulation, at which time progesterone synthesis increases (90). McNatty and colleagues (90) investigated the effects of prolactin on the secretion of progesterone by human ovarian granulosa cells *in vitro* in the presence of constant concentrations of LH and FSH. In the absence of prolactin, progesterone synthesis did not occur. However, in the presence of normal prolactin levels, progresterone synthesis did occur, although above a prolactin concentration of 20 ng/ml there was an inverse relationship between prolactin and progesterone (Fig. 4). The apparent block in progesterone synthesis by high prolactin levels could not be overcome by increasing the concentration of LH and FSH. Thus,

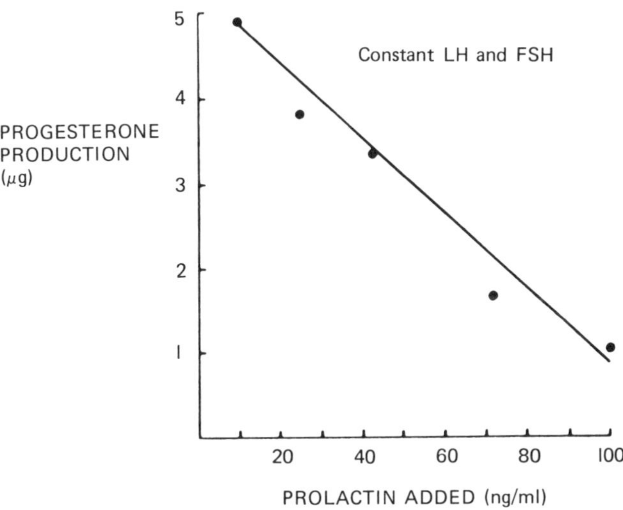

FIG. 4. Relationship between prolactin concentration and progesterone synthesis by human granulosa cells *in vitro*. (Modified with permission from McNatty et al., ref. 90.)

prolactin may modulate progesterone synthesis by the ovary but probably does not have a direct effect on estrogen synthesis.

Pharmacological elevation of prolactin levels with sulpiride in normal women leads to abolition of the progesterone rise in the luteal phase of the cycle and is followed by the development of amenorrhea (101). Furthermore, women with mild degrees of hyperprolactinemia may present with normal menstrual cycles but infertility; abnormal luteal phases have been documented in this setting (27,29). Lowering of prolactin levels to normal results in restoration of luteal function, with adequate progesterone synthesis (27,29). Administration of small doses of bromocriptine (1.5 mg b.i.d.) does not affect luteal function in normal women (26), but higher doses can lead to defective luteal function (106). Therefore, it is clear that prolactin deficiency caused by high doses of bromocriptine can lead to progesterone deficiency. Similarly, prolactin excess, either spontaneous or pharmacologically induced, will lead to defective luteal function (101).

In vivo studies in both women and men with hyperprolactinemia have demonstrated impaired gonadal steroid responses of the ovary and the testes to injections of exogenous gonadotropins (7,42). When prolactin levels were lowered to normal, the responsiveness of the gonad was restored. Similarly, Child and colleagues (19) reported a hyperprolactinemic patient in whom exogenous gonadotropin therapy was unsuccessful in inducing fertility. However, when her prolactin levels were restored to normal, spontaneous ovulation was restored.

Magrini and colleagues (88) investigated the effects of exogenous gonadotropins in normal men before and after prolactin levels were experimentally increased for 4 days with sulpiride. Plasma testosterone responses were the same, but the plasma dihydrotestosterone responses were impaired when the men were hyperprolactinemic. However, we were unable to demonstrate any change in circulating testosterone, dihydrotestosterone, or adrenal androgen levels under basal conditions or after human chorionic gonadotropin (hCG) stimulation during 4 weeks of hyperprolactinemia induced with metoclopramide in two normal men (119).

Furthermore, Carter and colleagues (15) were able to show neither resistance to the rise of testosterone to hCG in hyperprolactinemic men nor changes in response after prolactin levels were lowered to normal.

From the above it is clear that reduced gonadal function exists in association with hyperprolactinemia. The pathophysiology, however, is poorly defined. Several mechanisms may be involved, including defective gonadotropin secretion, abnormal positive feedback of estrogen, alterations in adrenal androgen secretion, and altered responses of the gonad to the gonadotropins.

VI. THERAPY FOR HYPERPROLACTINEMIA

A. Introduction

Hyperprolactinemia, if not the result of hypothyroidism, ingestion of psychotropic drugs, or section of the hypothalamo hypo physeal stalk, is usually the result of a pituitary adenoma. While such a neoplasm may be large (a macroadenoma), it is generally quite small (microadenoma). These tumors have been defined arbitrarily as macroadenomas or microadenomas if the diameter is greater than or less than 10 mm, respectively (69). Recognizing that both the patient and the physician feel more secure with a definite diagnosis, the practical value in deciding whether an individual patient has a microadenoma or idiopathic hyperprolactinemia is not as valuable as it might appear initially.

According to standard medical practice, the patient with a large pituitary tumor and visual field defects presents no dilemma; this patient requires surgical decompression. The remaining patients present a therapeutic challenge, since: (a) the natural history of micro- and macroadenomas is unknown; (b) the results of surgery in restoring normal hormonal secretion are variable; and (c) medical treatment is effective in suppressing prolactin levels to normal and restoring gonadal function and may also effect tumor growth *(see Chapter 7, page 154)*.

The aims of therapy should include: (a) reduction or removal of the tumor mass and reduction of its growth potential; (b) preservation of normal anterior pituitary function; and (c) reduction of prolactin levels to normal.

B. Making the Diagnosis of a Pituitary Tumor

The approach to diagnosis in an individual patient will include a thorough history and physical examination, which may provide clues as to the etiology of the hyperprolactinemia. Any patient with hyperprolactinemia requires expert neuroradiological examination. Often the pituitary fossa is normal or shows only subtle changes, such as sloping or dip of the floor on the anteroposterior view or a double contour or blister on the lateral view. Vezina and Sutton (127) have reported on the radiologic appearance of the sella in patients felt to have pituitary disease and have compared these findings with the actual tissue findings at the time of surgery. In two recent studies on the radiology of the pituitary fossa, the variations observed as a result of the asymmetry of the septum of the sphenoid sinus have been stressed. These may simulate an abnormality of the floor of the pituitary fossa (11,35). The delineation of the floor requires tomography, preferably the use of complex scanning.

It has been unequivocally demonstrated that abnormalities of the sella may be present that could easily have been missed on plain skull X-rays, and the use of tomography in all of these patients has been proposed (127). Tomography in two planes, using the hypocycloidal technique, detects minor changes that will be missed using plain X-rays alone.

A problem widely discussed and disputed by radiologists and endocrinologists relates to the criteria used to determine "normality" of the pituitary fossa; which radiologic abnormalities represent true disease and which are only normal variants (5,36)?

Besser (5) has stressed that studies of normal variants of the pituitary fossa have not been accompanied by endocrinologic evaluation of the patient. Since hyperprolactinemia is a common condition, it is conceivable that within a sample of 100 or 200 normal subjects a small number may have undiagnosed hyperprolactinemia, and this casts doubts on the validity of such studies (11, 35,110).

In a study of 80 patients with amenorrhea and galactorrhea, minor radiologic abnormalities of the pituitary fossa were seen in 64% with hyperprolactinemia, but abnormalities were also present in 36% of those with normal prolactin levels (2). Thus, Banna et al. (2) have concluded, "It is almost impossible to define a sharp line between the range of normal variation and minor pathological alteration."

To bring some objectivity into the assessment of the skull X-ray, both Vezina and Sutton (126) and Doyle and McLachlen (34) have proposed systems of grading the skull X-ray. Vezina and Sutton's system is unfortunately based on surgical results—the presence or absence of a breach of the cortex as seen at surgery. The classification of Doyle and McLachlen is descriptive, and we prefer it for that reason. This latter classification has been modified so that grade 0 is normal instead of grade 5, as in their classification (118). The presence or absence of a breach in the cortex of the bone has been treated as a separate criterion; if the cortex is breached, "E" is added as a suffix (Table 2).

The entire problem is compounded by the results of Costello's (23) study of 1,000 postmorten pituitaries from "normal" individuals, which demonstrated microadenomata in the pituitary in up to 21 to 22%. How many of these were functional and how many would have produced minor changes on skull X-ray? Kovacks and Ezrin (personal communication) consider the incidence of pituitary tumors in postmortem pituitaries to be no less than 10%, using current histological criteria of microadenomata, yet even that number makes this disease extremely common. A further series of 1,600 postmortem pituitaries indicated an incidence of 9.1% (89). Hardy, using the same criteria as those for the surgical specimens, reports an incidence of 2.6% (69).

The demonstration of a frank abnormality of the pituitary fossa on skull X-ray does not necessarily indicate that the fossa is full of tumor, since on pneumoencephalography air may be seen to enter the fossa, indicating "empty fossa syndrome" (cisternal herniation). This is seen in patients with hyperprolactinemia and, in our experience, is not infrequent (75a).

In view of our lack of knowledge about the natural history of the disease or the effects of various therapies on it, it is not possible to be dogmatic about a current approach to the problem. As discussed above, the patients with local symptoms from tumor present no dilemma, since surgical intervention is required.

In the patient with a normal skull X-ray, normal tomograms, and serum prolactin levels of less than 200 ng/ml, it is probably justifiable to proceed with medical therapy alone. In a patient with these findings who has a serum prolactin of greater than 200 ng/ml, the situation is more difficult. Statistically, this patient probably harbors a pituitary tumor. In general, there is a relationship between the pituitary tumor size and the level of prolactin (19,52,77,78,119). However, the results of surgical exploration of a radiologically normal pituitary fossa are frequently disap-

TABLE 2. *Classification of pituitary fossa on skull X-ray*

Grade	Lateral view	Posteroanterior view	Interpretation
B0	Single contour	Flat floor; no blistering	Normal
B1	<1 mm difference between contours	Minimal slope; <1 mm dip	Probably normal
B2	1–3 mm difference between contours; <3 mm blister	1–3 mm dip	Possibly abnormal
B3	>3 mm blister	Asymmetry >3 mm	Abnormal
B4	Double contour throughout	>3 mm asymmetry	Abnormal
B5	Both sides of fossa expanded in all directions (ballooned fossa)		Abnormal

Note: Presence of erosion of the sella turcica with breath of the cortex of bone is indicated by suffix E (e.g., **B2E**).

Modified from Doyle and McLachlan, ref. 34; reproduced with permission from Thorner et al., ref. 118.

pointing. Therefore, a trial of medical therapy with close follow-up may be the treatment of choice.

The desire for a pregnancy in a woman with hyperprolactinemia complicates the problem still further. The pituitary, in normal women, will increase 1½- to 2-fold during pregnancy (39). If a patient with a pituitary tumor—particularly a macroadenoma—is considering pregnancy, then prior treatment, either surgical or radiotherapeutic, aimed at reducing or removing the tumor is recommended by most investigators (12,19,47,59,75,117). Such treatment may significantly reduce the risk of tumor expansion during pregnancy, as well as the associated symptoms and signs, including headache, rise in intracranial pressure, and visual field defects. Of 14 hyperprolactinemic patients with radiologically abnormal fossae reported by Bergh et al. (4), who were not treated prior to pregnancy, 4 developed headaches and/or visual problems and demonstrable changes on skull X-ray during pregnancy. In contrast, Thorner and colleagues (119) reported on 82 pregnancies in 69 patients; 14 of these patients with frank pituitary tumors were previously treated with external pituitary irradiation and none developed visual symptoms or radiological changes suggestive of expansion of their tumors. Two other patients who had not received irradiation, as pregnancy was not planned, developed field defects.

C. Results of Surgical Treatment

Transsphenoidal surgery has advanced greatly in the past 15 years, with the advent of the operating microscope. Guiot and Hardy have pioneered the use of this technique in the treatment of hyperprolactinemia (66,69). In Hardy's hands the procedure has a very low morbidity and a high cure rate, particularly with noninvasive microadenomas (69). Many other groups are now using transsphenoidal surgery for the treatment of hyperprolactinemia, and published series reveal a wide range of results (17, 31,47,63,69,97,122,129) (Table 3). This disparity may reflect patient selection (97); the results in almost all series in which patients

TABLE 3. *Summary of published surgical results of treatment of hyperprolactinemia*

Reference	Evaluable patients	Prolactin lowered but not normalized	Prolactin normalized	Percent cured
17	23	14	11	49
47	9	9	7	78
63	10	4	6	60
69	80	—	59	74
122	36	34	24	67
129	24	23	8	33
31	71	—	17	24
96	30	30	21	70

were grouped by microadenoma or macroadenoma reflect very different results for the two conditions. In one series, the cure rate in patients with macroadenomas was only 15%, whereas in patients with microadenomas the cure rate was 56% (31). In another series, the figures were 0% and 59%, respectively (17). In contrast, Tindall and colleagues have reported good results for both microadenomas (71%) and macroadenomas (60%) (122).

The results reported by Hardy (69) represent the widest experience of the use of transsphenoidal surgery and probably reflect the optimum that can be achieved at present. In patients with localized microadenomas the cure rate, as defined by normalization of prolactin, was 90%; in those patients with enclosed adenomas (including 7 with suprasellar extension) the cure rate was 53%; in those patients with invasive adenomas the cure rate was 43%; and in the 1 patient in whom the fossa had been entirely destroyed, the prolactin was lowered but not into the normal range. Even in the best hands, the patients with readily identifiable microadenomas are the only ones in whom there can be preoperative confidence that cure may be obtained by surgery alone.

However, a problem that endocrinologists encounter in assessing the results of surgery is that very few series report on full assessment of endocrinologic testing in their patients before surgery and more importantly, postoperatively. Documentation of the reserve of ACTH, growth hormone (during hypoglycemia), TSH (after TRH), and gonadotropins is necessary, together with normalization of prolactin levels. Furthermore, return of menses is only one parameter of gonadal function in women; the ultimate proof would be conception. If pregnancy is not desired, an adequate progesterone rise in the luteal phase of the cycle should be documented. Similarly, testosterone levels and seminal analyses should be performed in men. It is therefore impossible to assess the true incidence of hypopituitarism induced by surgery at this time, although some figures suggest it may be as high as 25% (130).

From these data it would appear that the aims of surgery using the transsphenoidal approach should be to cure patients with localized, noninvasive microadenomas and to decompress invasive tumors, primarily to reduce the risk of tumor expansion. Medical therapy can then be added to lower prolactin levels to normal.

D. Results of Radiation Therapy

External pituitary irradiation has been used for many years, with some success in the treatment of nonfunctioning pituitary tumors and in those that secrete ACTH and growth hormone (95,103). In general, pituitary irradiation arrests the tumor growth and often lowers the circulating levels of the tumor product. The major disadvantage of irradiation is that it may take up to 5 or more years to become maximally effective. Irradiation carries a very low morbidity. Relatively few data are available on the results of irradiation of prolactinomas. Reyes and colleagues (100) reported on 7 patients treated with external pituitary irradiation alone. Although only 1 became normoprolactinemic, local symptoms from the tumor improved in 3 patients with these symptoms, menses resumed in 4, galactorrhea was reduced in all, and remineralization of the pituitary fossa was seen in all 5 patients following 1 year of treatment. Our own results are difficult to evaluate, since all but 1 patient were coincidentally started on bromocriptine. In this one individual, galactorrhea has ceased and prolactin levels have progressively fallen, although not to normal. Other approaches to irradiation have been used in patients with hyperprolactinemia and pituitary tumors. Included is implantation of radioactive yttrium, but results appear to be similar to those described above for external pituitary irradiation, with a lowering of prolactin levels to approximately 40% of those seen before treatment, but not a lowering to normal. Supplementation with medical therapy has been required in most instances to restore fertility (19,77). Heavy particle irradiation is also now being applied to patients with hyperprolactinemia (79). However, the long-term effects of this form of therapy on pituitary function are not known.

E. Medical Therapy

Medical therapy, therefore, has a clear role, either as the primary therapy in patients without frank tumors, or as an adjunct to partially successful surgery or radiotherapy that leaves the patient hyperprolactinemic. The choice of therapy in an individual patient depends not only on his prolactin levels and skull X-ray, but also on the expertise, surgical or radiotherapeutic, at a given center.

The ergot alkaloids, as discussed in Chapter 2, are potent drugs with a host of pharmacological effects. Bromocriptine was developed specifically as an inhibitor of prolactin secretion (43). It was only several years after its introduction into clinical practice that it was discovered to be a dopamine receptor stimulant (dopamine agonist) (22,56). Since it is now widely agreed that dopamine is one, if not the most important, prolactin inhibiting factor, bromocriptine may be considered to act as an analog of endogenous dopamine. This compound was selected because, in contrast to ergocryptine, it has only very weak cardiovascular and oxytocic effects. It also has advantages over levodopa, since it does not need to be converted to dopamine to be effective and is relatively specific for the dopamine receptor *(see Chapter 2, p. 31)*. Furthermore, it has a long duration of action. This characteristic is well illustrated *in vitro* (132), using isolated rat anterior pituitary cells, where its effect persists for greater than 3 hr after its withdrawal (Fig. 5). The acute effects in 18 hyperprolactinemic women of a single 2.5 mg oral dose of bromocriptine are seen in Fig. 6. The effects were delayed for 1 hr, after which inhibition of prolactin release was observed. Bromocriptine levels of 0.46 ng/ml were observed at 1 hr, and at 3 hr peak levels of 0.76 ng/ml were seen. In spite of falling levels of the drug, prolactin suppression was maintained for the subsequent 8 hr. Thus, its long duration

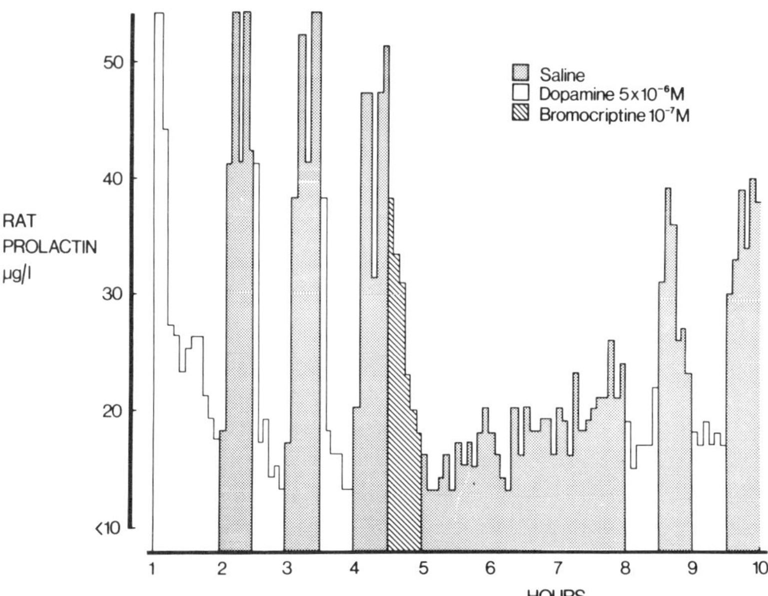

FIG. 5. Prolactin concentration in eluate from pituitary cell column demonstrating the slower onset of inhibition of prolactin release by bromocriptine (10^{-7} M) than dopamine (5×10^{-6} M) and its long duration of action after withdrawal. (Reproduced with permission from Yeo et al., ref. 132.)

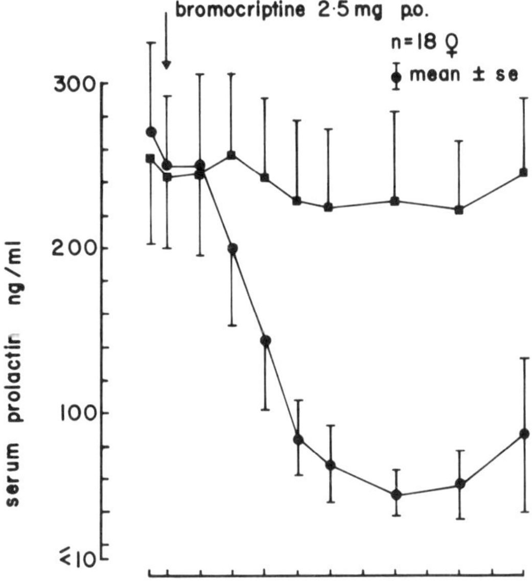

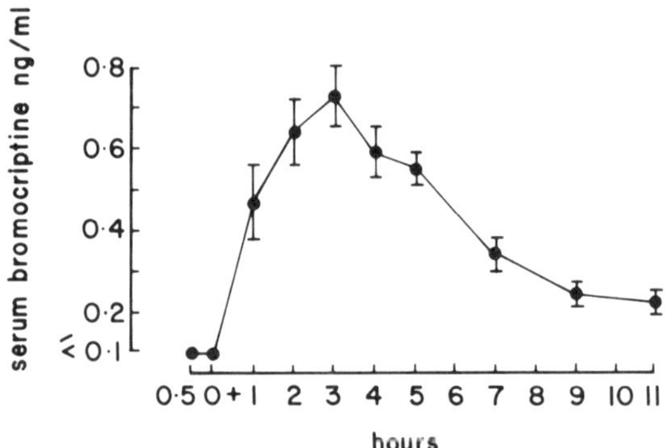

FIG. 6. Mean (± SEM) serum prolactin and bromocriptine levels in 18 hyperprolactinemic women during a control study and after bromocriptine 2.5 mg p.o. at 0 hours. (Reproduced with permission from Thorner et al., ref. 120.)

of action at the lactotroph is observed *in vivo* as well. The normal dose of 2.5 mg b.i.d. or t.i.d. is adequate to keep prolactin levels suppressed throughout the day (Fig. 7).

Bromocriptine therapy should be initiated in slowly increasing doses and during meals; in this way, the side effects of nausea, vomiting, and postural hypotension, which are sometimes seen at the beginning of therapy, are avoided *(see Chapter 6).* On retiring, 1.25 or 2.5 mg is taken. Each 2 to 4 days the dose is increased by 2.5 mg until 2.5 mg b.i.d. or t.i.d. is achieved. This dose is usually sufficient to lower prolactin levels to normal, but occasionally it may be necessary to increase the dose to 15 to 30 mg/day in divided doses.

1. Results of Bromocriptine Treatment in Women

Galactorrhea decreases within a few days or weeks of the start of bromocriptine therapy. Normal menstrual cycles, with ovulation, are rapidly restored in the majority of patients (Fig. 8). Usually, patients who are suspected to have pituitary tumors on the basis of their skull X-rays take longer for their cycles to be restored (115).

In our series of 36 patients with idiopathic hyperprolactinemia, 40% had restoration of cycles within 1 month, and by 2 months this figure was greater than 80%. Of 26 women with suspected pituitary tumors, periods were restored in 22. Of the 4 who remained amenorrheic, 3 had been treated previously with transfrontal surgery and radiotherapy. Other groups have had similarly gratifying results (28,53,78). Our most recent results at the University of Virginia reflect the same pattern (120). In this series, special care was taken to document normal luteal function. Of 18 women with hyperprolactinemia and amenorrhea, cycles were restored in 15, and in 13 patients normal luteal function was documented by pregnancy, or by a normal rise in serum progesterone and/or a secretory endometrium on endometrial biopsy.

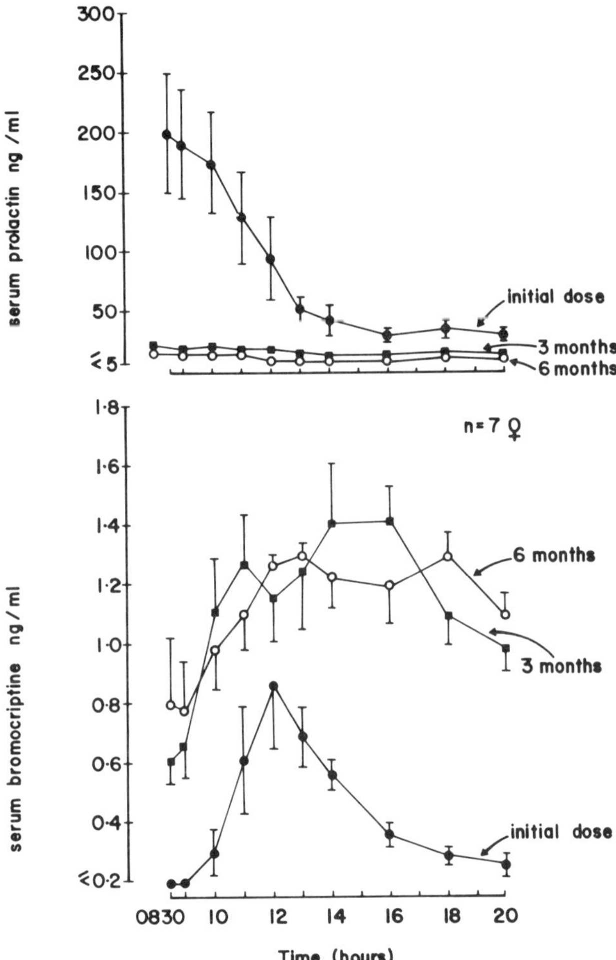

FIG. 7. Mean (± SEM) serum prolactin and bromocriptine levels in 7 hyperprolactinemic women after their initial oral dose of 2.5 mg bromocriptine and at 3 months and 6 months on bromocriptine 2.5 mg t.i.d. (Reproduced with permission from Thorner et al., ref. 120.)

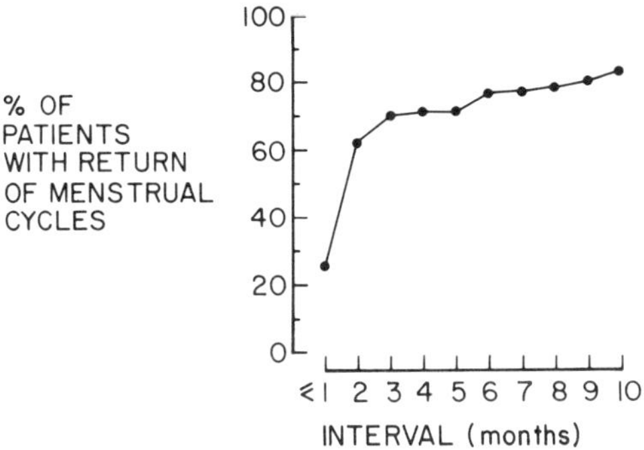

FIG. 8. Cumulative percentage of 58 amenorrheic hyperprolactinemic women with return of regular menstrual cycles related to months on bromocriptine therapy.

2. *Pregnancy and Bromocriptine*

Many women present initially with infertility; for them, the goal of therapy is pregnancy. At this time, bromocriptine is permitted for use in the United States only for short periods of time, and patients are required by the FDA recommendations to use contraceptive precautions. However, in a large number of countries, including Canada and many in western Europe, the drug is approved by the licensing authorities for the treatment of infertility associated with hyperprolactinemia. In the past, these patients have classically been treated with clomiphene or exogenous gonadotropins. Clomiphene is generally ineffective (96), and exogenous gonadotropins carry the potentially catastrophic risks of overstimulation syndrome of the ovary and multiple pregnancy.

We have previously discussed some of the potential risks of pregnancy in hyperprolactinemic patients, the most serious of which is the risk of swelling of any pituitary tumor during pregnancy (117,119). As noted above *(p. 77)*, the probability of this occurring is small—probably less than 5% in patients with microadenomas and up to 35% in macroadenomas (59). The swelling may possibly be avoided by prior treatment of the tumor with external irradiation and/or surgery before pregnancy. However, Griffith et al. (65) reported tumor expansion in only 9 of 116 completed pregnancies in patients with pituitary tumors. However, it should be recognized that the same risks pertain in those patients with pituitary tumors whose fertility is restored by other means, such as exogenous gonadotropins.

A further risk, stressed in the American literature, is the possibility of teratogenic effects of bromocriptine. At present, according to 805 pregnancies documented by Sandoz (Table 4), there does not appear to be an increased risk of fetal malformations. However, until the numbers are larger and the children born to women who conceived while on bromocriptine have lived their complete life cycle, no definitive statement can be made. It can only be stated that to date there are no data suggesting that the drug has teratogenic effects (64). Furthermore, this therapy is far more convenient and physiological than exogenous

TABLE 4. *Outcome of 805 pregnancies in women treated with bromocriptine*

		Expected incidence
Total pregnancies	805	
Spontaneous abortion	97	81–202
Induced abortion	22	
Missed abortion	6	
Extrauterine pregnancy	7	
Hydatiform mole	2	
Twins	16	10
Triplets	1	
Singletons	654	
Total live babies	689	
Congenital abnormalities	20	15
Major: pulmonary atresia	1	
renal agenesis	1	
Down's syndrome	1	
reduction deformities	3	
hip dislocation	5	
Minor	9	

From Dr. R. L. Elton, Sandoz, Inc., *personal communication.*

gonadotropin therapy and does not carry the risk of multiple ovulation, nor does it require daily monitoring of blood or urine to prevent the ovarian hyperstimulation syndrome. These conclusions have been confirmed in our combined experience of some 100 pregnancies at St. Bartholomew's Hospital in London and at the University of Virginia.

3. Results of Bromocriptine Treatment in Men

Hyperprolactinemia in men is much less common than in women and is more often associated with macroadenomas. Many of these patients have multiple anterior pituitary hormone deficiencies (6,15,48,92,114–116). Impotence and diminished libido are frequently noted; serum testosterone levels are generally low. Of interest is the fact that testosterone replacement therapy in these patients often fails to restore libido and potency (15).

As discussed above, the mechanism by which hyperprolactinemia leads to hypogonadism in both men and women is not clear. Furthermore, although in some patients testosterone levels rise during bromocriptine therapy, in others potency is restored before there is any change in testosterone levels (48). Thus, the restoration of sexual functions may be a direct effect on neuronal mechanisms by bromocriptine or of the lowering of prolactin levels, rather than being related to other indirect hormonal events, such as an increase in testosterone levels. Finally, bromocriptine results in cessation of galactorrhea if present, but this symptom is far less common in men than in women.

4. Withdrawal of Bromocriptine Treatment

Bromocriptine is effective in maintaining suppression of prolactin secretion for the duration of therapy. In general, it has been our experience that circulating prolactin levels return to their pretreatment levels following withdrawal of therapy (Fig. 9). Recently, Von Werder and colleagues (128) reported that after several years of bromocriptine therapy, prolactin levels do not rise

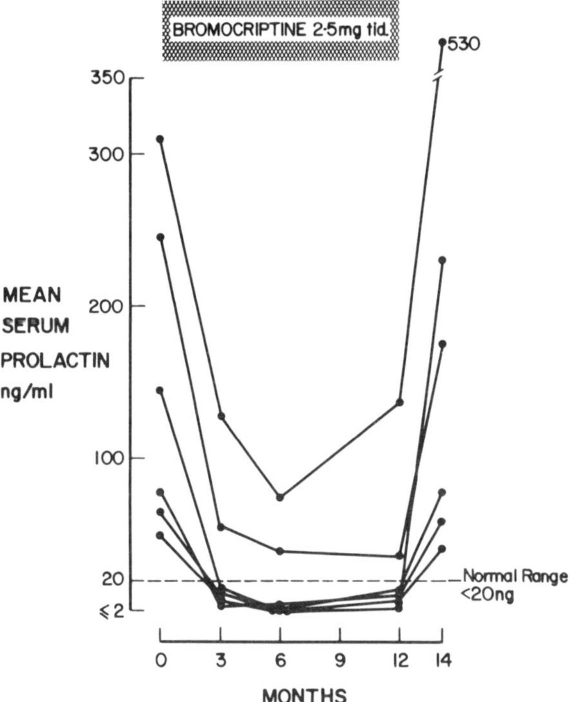

FIG. 9. Mean serum prolactin levels of 10 samples drawn through the day in 6 hyperprolactinemic women prior to, and at 3, 6, and 12 months during 2.5 mg t.i.d. bromocriptine therapy and 2 months after withdrawal.

to pretreatment levels following withdrawal of therapy. However, it was not clear how many of their patients had also had irradiation; therefore, the results are difficult to interpret. It is clear that bromocriptine therapy can reduce tumor size in some patients with large pituitary tumors. This is discussed in detail in Chapter 7.

Although bromocriptine is only approved for short-term use in the United States, in other countries it is used in long-term therapy for hyperprolactinemia. Several patients have been on continuous therapy for 9 years without evidence of adverse effects.

If therapy is continued on a long-term basis, it is probably advisable to withdraw patients from therapy for 2 months every 1 to 2 years to confirm that their prolactin levels rise when treatment is withheld.

VII. SUPPRESSION OF PHYSIOLOGICAL LACTATION WITH BROMOCRIPTINE

In Europe, the United States, and many other parts of the western world, many women choose not to breast feed their babies. Furthermore, women who give birth to stillborn infants, who undergo spontaneous or therapeutic abortion, or those in whom there is a medical contraindication to lactation often need an effective method for suppression of lactation.

The process of lactation depends on three stages: (a) *mammogenesis*—the growth of the mammary gland at puberty, which is completed during pregnancy; (b) *lactogenesis*—initiation of milk secretion, which occurs after delivery; and (c) *galactopoiesis*—the maintenance of established lactation. Lactogenesis and galactopoiesis are dependent on a large number of hormones, but prolactin is essential for both. Suppression of lactation has in the past been achieved by mechanical means (binding the breast), by fluid restriction and diuretics, or by the administration of estrogens. Estrogens block the effects of prolactin at the level of the breast but also stimulate prolactin secretion from the pituitary. The logical approach to achieve suppression of lactation would be to suppress prolactin secretion (20,102,125). Bromocriptine has been used for this purpose and is extremely effective, not only in lowering prolactin levels to normal but also in preventing initiation or maintenance of lactation. In several double-blind studies (10,102,123) it has been shown to be superior to estrogens and to have the advantage of not affecting the blood clotting system. Therefore, it is not associated with an increased risk of deep vein thrombosis or thromboembolism, as occurs with estrogens (20).

Bromocriptine, 2.5 mg, is administered orally at time of delivery and continued at a dose of 2.5 mg twice daily for 2 weeks, with a further week of a once-daily regimen to prevent rebound lactation. In postpartum women, bromocriptine therapy is not associated with side effects. It is also effective in suppression of established lactation.

VIII. CONCLUSIONS

Hyperprolactinemia is probably the most common hypothalamic–pituitary disease. Hyperprolactinemic patients may present with symptoms from their endocrine disturbance—usually galactorrhea and/or hypogonadism—or with symptoms from expansion of their pituitary tumor. Therapy directed at removing or destroying any pituitary tumor does not always result in restoration of circulating prolactin levels to normal or return of normal gonadal function. However, medical therapy with bromocriptine, which acts by stimulating pituitary dopamine receptors, results in lowering of prolactin levels, usually to normal, even in patients with pituitary tumors. It is effective in restoring gonadal function and fertility. Bromocriptine may also suppress growth of prolactin-secreting tumors. It is the treatment of choice for suppression of puerperal lactation and lactation following abortion.

REFERENCES

1. Armstrong, D. T., Knudsen, K. A., and Miller, L. S. (1970): Effects of prolactin upon cholesterol metabolism and progesterone biosynthesis in corpora lutea of rats hypophysectomized during pseudopregnancy. *Endocrinology,* 86:634–641.
2. Banna, M., Nicholas, W., and McLachelin, M. (1978): The borderline pituitary fossa in patients with amenorrhoea and for galactorrhoea. *Neuroradiology,* 16:440–442.
3. Ben David, M., Danon, A., Benveniste, R., Weller, C. P., and Sulman, P. G. (1971): Results of radioimmunoassays of rat pituitary and serum prolactin after adenalectomy and perphenazine treatment in rats. *J. Endocrinol.,* 50:599–606.
4. Bergh, T., Nillius, S., and Wide, L. (1978): Clinical course and outcome of pregnancies in amenorrheic women with hyperprolactinemia and pituitary tumours. *Br. Med. J.,* 1:875–880.

5. Besser, G. M. (1976): The pituitary fossa—Normal or abnormal? *Br. J. Radiol.,* 49:652–653.
6. Besser, G. M., Parkes, L., Edwards, C. R. W., Forsyth, I. A., and McNeilly, A. S. (1972): Galactorrhoea: Successful treatment with reduction of plasma prolactin levels by brom-ergocryptine. *Br. Med. J.,* 3:669–672.
7. Besser, G. M., and Thorner, M. O. (1976): Bromocriptine in the treatment of the hyperprolactinaemia-hypogonadism syndromes. *Postgrad. Med. J.,* 52 (Suppl. 1):64–70.
8. Bohnet, H. G., Dahlen, H. G., Wuttke, W., and Schneider, H. P. G. (1976): Hyperprolactinaemic anovulatory syndrome. *J. Clin. Endocrinol. Metab.,* 42:132–143.
9. Boyar, R. M., Kapen, S., Finkelstein, J. W., Perlow, M., Sassin, J. F., Fukushima, D. K., Weitzman, E. D., and Hellman, L. (1974): Hypothalamic-pituitary function in diverse hyperprolactinemic states. *J. Clin. Invest.,* 53:1588–1598.
10. Brun, del Re, R., del Pozo, E., de Grandi, P., Friesen, H., Hinselmann, M., and Wyss, H. (1973): Prolactin inhibition and suppression of puerperal lactation by a Br-ergocryptine (CB 154). A comparison with estrogen. *Obstet. Gynecol.,* 41:884–890.
11. Bruneton, J. N., Drouillard, J. P., Sabatier, J. C., Elie, G. P., and Tavernier, J. F. (1979): Normal variants of the sella turcica. *Radiology,* 131:99–104.
12. Burke, C. W., Joplin, G. P., and Fraser, R. (1972): Pituitary tumour treated by pituitary implantation of yttrium 90 during or before pregnancy (two cases). *Proc. R. Soc. Med.,* 65:486–488.
13. Calabro, M., and MacLeod, R. M. (1978): Binding of dopamine to bovine anterior pituitary gland membranes. *Neuroendocrinology,* 25:32–46.
14. Caron, M. C., Beaulieu, M., Raymond, V., Gagne, B., Drouin, J., Lefkowitz, R. J., and Labrie, F. (1978): Dopaminergic receptors in the anterior pituitary gland. *J. Biol. Chem.,* 253:2244–2253.
15. Carter, J. N., Tyson, J. E., Tolis, G., Van Vliet, S., Faiman, C., and Friesen, H. G. (1978): Prolactin-secreting tumors and hypogonadism in 22 men. *N. Engl. J. Med.,* 299:847–852.
16. Carter, J. N., Tyson, J. E., Warne, G. L., McNeilly, A. S., Faiman, C., and Friesen, H. G. (1977): Adrenocortical function in hyperprolactinemic women. *J. Clin. Endocrinol. Metab.,* 45:973–980.
17. Chang, R. J., Keye, W. R., Jr., Young, J. R., Wilson, C. B., and Jaffe, R. B. (1977): Detection, evaluation, and treatment of pituitary microadenomas in patients with galactorrhea and amenorrhea. *Am. J. Obstet. Gynecol.,* 128:356–363.
18. Chester Jones, I., Phillips, J. G., and Bellamy, D. (1962): Studies on water and electrolytes in cyclostomes and teleosts with special reference to myxine *glutinosa L.* (the hagfish) and *Anguilla anguilla L.* (the Atlantic eel). *Gen. Comp. Endocrinol.,* Suppl. 1:36–47.
19. Child, D. F., Gordon, H., Mashiter, K., and Joplin, G. F. (1975): Pregnancy, prolactin and pituitary tumors. *Br. Med. J.,* 4:87–89.
20. Cooke, I., Jenkins, A., Foley, M., Obiekwe, B., Lenton, E., McNeilly, A., Preston, E., Parsons, J., Millar, D., and Kennedy, G. (1976): The

treatment of puerperal lactation with bromocriptine. *Postgrad. Med. J.*, 52 (Suppl. 1):75–80.
21. Copinshi, G., L'Hermite, M., Leclercq, R., Goldstein, J., Vanhaelst, L., Virasore, E., and Robyn, C. (1975): Effects of glucocorticoids on pituitary hormonal responses to hypoglycemia. Inhibition of prolactin release. *J. Clin. Endocrinol. Metab.*, 40:442–449.
22. Corrodi, H., Fuxe, K., Hokfelt, T., Lidbrink, P., and Ungerstedt, U. (1973): Effect of ergot drugs on central catecholamine neurons: Evidence for a stimulation of central dopamine neurons. *J. Pharm. Pharmacol.*, 25:409–412.
23. Costello, R. T. (1936): Subclinical adenoma of the pituitary gland. *Am. J. Pathol.*, 12:205–215.
24. Coulam, C., Annegers, J. F., Abboud, C. F., Laws, E. R., and Kurland, L. T. (1979): Pituitary adenoma and oral contraceptives: A case-control study. *Fertil. Steril.*, 31:25–28.
25. Cronin, M. J., Roberts, J. M., and Weiner, R. I. (1978): Dopamine and dihydroergocryptine binding to the anterior pituitary and other brain areas of the rat and sheep. *Endocrinology*, 103:302–309.
25a. Cronin, M. J., Cheung, C. Y., Wilson, C. B., Monroe, S. E., Jaffe, R. B., and Weiner, R. I. (1980): ^{3}H-Spiperone binding to human anterior pituitaries and pituitary adenomas secreting prolactin, growth hormone and ACTH. *J. Clin. Endocrinol. Metab. (in press).*
26. Del Pozo, E., Goldstein, M., Friesen, H., Brun, del Re, R., and Eppenberger, U. (1975): Lack of prolactin suppression on the regulation of the human menstrual cycle. *Am. J. Obstet. Gynecol.*, 123:719–723.
27. Del Pozo, E., and Lancranjan, I. (1978): Clinical use of drugs modifying the release of anterior pituitary hormones. In: *Frontiers in Neuroendocrinology*, Vol. 5, edited by W. F. Ganong and L. Martini, pp. 207–247. Raven Press, New York.
28. Del Pozo, E., Varga, L., Wyss, H., Tolis, G., Friesen, H., Wenner, R., Vetter, L., and Uettwiler, A. (1974): Clinical and hormonal response to bromocriptine (CB 154) in the galactorrhoea syndromes. *J. Clin. Endocrinol. Metab.*, 39:18–26.
29. Del Pozo, E., Wyss, H., Lancranjan, I., Obolensley, W., and Varga, L. (1976): Prolactin induced luteal insufficiency and its treatment with bromocriptine: Preliminary results. In: *Ovulation in the Human*, edited by P. G. Crosignani and D. R. Mishell, pp. 297–299. Academic Press, London.
30. Delvoye, P., Demaegd, M., Uwayitu-Nyampeta, and Robyn, C. (1978): Serum prolactin, gonadotropins and estradiol in menstruating and amenorrheic mothers during two years' lactation. *Am. J. Obstet. Gynecol.*, 130:635–639.
31. Derome, P. J., Peillon, F., Bard, R. H., Jedynak, C. P., Racadot, J., and Guiot, G. (1979): Adenomes a prolactine: Resultats du traitment chirugical. *Nouv. Presse Med.*, 8:577–583.
32. Desphande, N. (1975): Regulation of androgen synthesis in the human adrenal gland *in vivo* and *in vitro. Horm. Res.*, 6:294–295.

33. Douglas, W. W., and Taraskevich, P. S. (1978): Action potentials in gland cells of rat pituitary pars intermedia: Inhibition by dopamine, an inhibitor of MSH secretion. *J. Physiol.,* 285:171–184.
34. Doyle, F., and McLachlan, M. (1977): Radiological aspects of pituitary-hypothalamic disease. *J. Clin. Endocrinol. Metabol.,* 6:53–81.
35. Dubois, P. J., Orr, D. P., Hoy, R. J., Herbert, D. L., and Heinz, E. R. (1979): Normal sellar variations in frontal tomograms. *Radiology,* 131:105–110.
36. Du Boulay, G. (1976): The pituitary fossa—Normal or abnormal. *Br. J. Radiol.,* 49:653.
37. Dupont, A., and Redding, T. W. (1975): Purification and characterization of PIF from pig hypothalami. *Program 57th Meeting of the Endocrine Society,* New York, Abstract 85.
38. Enjalbert, A., Moos, F., Carbonell, L., Priam, M., and Kordon, C. (1977): Prolactin inhibiting activity of dopamine—Free subcellular fractions from rat mediobasal hypothalamus. *Neuroendocrinology,* 24:147–161.
39. Erdheim, J., and Stumme, E. (1909): Ubere die schwangerschaftsveranderung der hypophyse. *Beitr. Pathol. Anat.,* 46:1–132.
40. Evans, W. S., Rogol, A. D., MacLeod, R. M., and Thorner, M. O. (1980): Dopaminergic mechanisms and LH secretion: I. Acute administration of the dopamine agonist bromocriptine does not inhibit LH release in hyperprolactinemic women. *J. Clin. Endocrinol. Metab.,* 50:103–107.
41. Everett, J. W. (1954): The luteotrophic function of autografts of the rat hypophysis. *Endocrinology,* 54:685–690.
42. Faglia, G., Beck-Peccoz, P., Travaglini, P., Ambrosi, B., Rondena, M., Paracchi, A., Spada, A., Weber, G., Bara, R., and Bouzin, A. (1977): Functional studies in hyperprolactinemic states. In: *Prolactin and Human Reproduction.* edited by P. G. Crosignani and C. Robyn, pp. 225–238. Academic Press, New York.
43. Flückiger, E., and Wagner, H. (1968): 2-Br-α-ergokryptin: Beeinflussung von fertilität und laktation bei der ratte. *Experientia,* 24:1130–1131.
44. Forbes, A. P., Henneman, P. H., Griswold, G. C., and Albright, F. (1954): Syndrome characterized by galactorrhea, amenorrhea and low urinary FSH: Comparison with acromegaly and normal lactation. *J. Clin. Endocrinol. Metab.,* 14:265–271.
45. Forsyth, I. A., Besser, G. M., Edwards, C. R. W., Francis, L., and Myres, R. P. (1971): Plasma prolactin activity in inappropriate lactation. *Br. Med. J.,* 3:225–227.
46. Forsyth, I. A., and Myres, R. P. (1971): Human prolactin. Evidence obtained by the bioassay of human plasma. *J. Endocrinol.,* 51:157–168.
47. Franks, S., Jacobs, H. S., Hull, M. G. R., Steele, S. J., and Nabarro, J. D. N. (1977): Management of hyperprolactinemic amenorrhea. *Br. J. Obstet. Gynaecol.,* 84:241–253.
48. Franks, S., Jacobs, H. S., Martin, N., and Nabarro, J. D. N. (1978): Hyperprolactinemia and impotence. *Clin. Endocrinol. (Oxf.),* 8:277–287.
49. Franks, S., Murray, M. A. F., Jequier, A. M., Steele, S. J., Nabarro,

J. D. N., and Jacobs, H. S. (1975): Incidence and significance of hyperprolactinemia in women with amenorrhea. *Clin. Endocrinol. (Oxf.)*, 4:597–607.

50. Franks, S., Nabarro, J. D. N., and Jacobs, H. S. (1977): Prevalence and presentation of hyperprolactinemia in patients with "functionless" pituitary tumors. *Lancet*, 1:778–780.
51. Frantz, A. G., and Kleinberg, D. L. (1970): Prolactin: Evidence that it is separate from growth hormone in human blood. *Science*, 170:745–746.
52. Friesen, H. G. (1978): Human prolactin. *Ann. R. Coll. Physicians Surg. Can.*, 11:275–281.
53. Friesen, H. G., and Tolis, G. (1977): The use of bromocriptine in the galactorrhea amenorrhea syndromes. The Canadian Co-operative study. *Clin. Endocrinol. (Oxf.)*, 6 (Suppl):91–99s.
54. Frohman, L. A., and Szabo, M. (1975): Evidence for the existence of prolactin releasing activity distinct from TRH in passive hypothalamic extracts. *Program 57th Annual Meeting of the Endocrine Society*, New York, Abstract 86.
55. Furth, J., Gadsden, E. L., Clifton, K. H., and Anderson, E. (1956): Autonomous mammatropic pituitary tumors in mice. Their somatotropic features and responsiveness to estrogens. *Cancer Res.*, 16:600–607.
56. Fuxe, K., Corrodi, H., Hökfelt, T., Lidbrink, P., and Ungerstedt, U. (1974): Ergocornine and 2-Br-α-ergocryptine. Evidence for prolonged dopamine receptor stimulation. *Med. Biol.*, 52:121–132.
57. Fuxe, K., Hökfelt, A., Löfström, A., Johansson, O., Agnati, L., Everitt, B., Goldstein, M., Jeffcoate, S., White, N., Eneroth, P., Gustafsson, J.-A., and Skett, P. (1976): On the role of neurotransmitters and hypothalamic hormones and their interactions in hypothalamic and extrahypothalamic control of pituitary function and sexual behavior. In: *Subcellular Mechanisms in Reproductive Neuroendocrinology*, edited by F. Naftolin, K. J. Ryan, and I. J. Davies, pp. 193–246. Elsevier, Amsterdam.
58. Gautvick, K. M., Tashjian, A. H., Jr., Kourides, I. A., Weintraub, B. D., Graeber, C. T., Maloof, F., Suzuki, K., and Zuckerman, J. E. (1974): Thyrotropin-releasing hormone, prolactin and suckling. *N. Engl. J. Med.*, 290:1162–1165.
59. Gemzell, C., and Wang, C. F. (1979): Outcome of pregnancy in women with pituitary adenomas. *Fertil. Steril.*, 31:363–372.
60. Gibbs, D. M., and Neill, J. D. (1978): Dopamine levels in hypophyseal stalk blood in the rat are sufficient to inhibit prolactin secretion *in vivo*. *Endocrinology*, 102:1895–1900.
61. Giusti, G., Bassi, F., Forti, G., Giannotti, P., Calabresi, E., Pazzagli, M., Fiorelli, G., Mannelli, M., Misciglia, N., and Serio, M. (1977): Effects of prolactin on androgen secretion by the human adrenal cortex. In: *Progress in Prolactin Physiology and Pathology*, edited by C. Robyn and M. Harter, pp. 293–303. Elsevier, Amsterdam.
62. Glass, M. R., Shaw, R. W., Butt, W. R., Logan Edwards, R., and London, D. R. (1975): An abnormality of oestrogen feedback in amenorrhea galactorrhea. *Br. Med. J.*, 111:274–275.

63. Gomez, F., Reyes, F. I., and Faiman, C. (1977): Nonpuerperal galactorrhea and hyperprolactinemia. *Am. J. Med.*, 62:648–660.
64. Griffith, R. W., Turkalj, I., and Braun, P. (1978): Outcome of pregnancy in mothers given bromocriptine. *Br. J. Clin. Pharmacol.*, 5:227–231.
65. Griffith, R. W., Turkalj, I., and Braun, P. (1979): Pituitary tumours during pregnancy in mothers treated with bromocriptine. *Br. J. Clin. Pharmacol.*, 7:393–396.
66. Guiot, G. (1973): Transsphenoidal approach in surgical treatment of pituitary adenomas: General principles and indications in non-functioning adenomas. In: *Diagnosis and Treatment of Pituitary Tumors; Proceedings of a Conference,* edited by P. O. Kohler and G. T. Ross, pp. 159–178. American Elsevier, New York.
67. Guyda, H., Hwang, P., and Friesen, H. (1971): Immunologic evidence for monkey and human prolactin (MPr and HPr). *J. Clin. Endocrinol. Metab.*, 32:120–123.
68. Haeusler, G. (1972): Differential effect of verapamil on excitation-contraction coupling in smooth muscle and on excitation-secretion coupling in adrenergic nerve terminals. *J. Pharmacol. Exp. Ther.*, 180:672–682.
68a. Hall, R., Anderson, J., Smart, G. A., Besser, G. M. (1974): *Fundamentals of Clinical Endocrinology.* Pitman Medical, London.
69. Hardy, J., Beauregard, H., and Robert, F. (1978): Prolactin-secreting pituitary adenomas: Transsphenoidal microsurgical treatment. In: *Progress in Prolactin Physiology and Pathology,* edited by C. Robyn and M. Harter, pp. 361–370. American Elsevier, New York.
70. Hoff, J. D., Lasley, B. K., Wang, C. F., and Yen, S. S. C. (1973): The two pools of pituitary gonadotropin: Regulation during the menstrual cycle. *J. Clin. Endocrinol. Metab.*, 44:302–312.
71. Hwang, P., Guyda, H., and Friesen, H. (1971): A radioimmunoassay for human prolactin. *Proc. Soc. Natl. Acad. Sci. (U.S.A.),* 68:1902–1906.
72. Ingvarson, C. G. (1969): The action of prolactin on the adrenocortical function. *Acta Rheumatol. Scand.*, 15:18–20.
73. Jacobs, H. S., Franks, S., Murray, M. A. F., Hull, M. G. R., Steele, S. J., and Nabarro, J. D. N. (1976): Clinical and endocrine features of hyperprolactinemic amenorrhoea. *Clin. Endocrinol. (Oxf.),* 5:439–454.
74. Jacobs, H. S., Knuth, U. A., Hull, M. G. R., and Franks, S. (1977): Post-"pill" amenorrhoea—Cause or coincidence. *Br. Med. J.*, 2:940–942.
75. Jewelewicz, R., Zimmerman, E. A., and Carmel, P. W. (1977): Conservative management of a pituitary tumor during pregnancy following induction of ovulation with gonadotropins. *Fertil. Steril.*, 28:35–40.
75a. Jordan, R. M., Kendall, J. W., and Kerber, C. W. (1977): The primary empty sella syndrome. Analysis of the clinical characteristics, radiographic features, pituitary function and cerebrospinal fluid adenohypophyseal hormone concentrations. *Am. J. Med.*, 62:569–580.
76. Judd, S. J., Rakoff, J. S., and Yen, S. S. C. (1978): Inhibition of gonadotropin and prolactin release by dopamine: Effect of endogenous estradiol levels. *J. Clin. Endocrinol. Metab.*, 47:494–498.
77. Kelly, W. F., Mashiter, K., Doyle, F. H., Banks, L. M., and Joplin,

G. F. (1978): Treatment of prolactin-secreting pituitary tumours in young women by needle implantation of radioactive yttrium. *Q. J. Med.*, 47:473–493.

78. Kleinberg, D. L., Noel, G. L., and Frantz, A. G. (1977): Galactorrhea: 235 cases including 48 with pituitary tumors. *N. Engl. J. Med.*, 296:589–600.
79. Kliman, B., and Kjellberg, R. N. (1977): Proton beam therapy of pituitary tumors in women with galactorrhea, amenorrhea, and elevated serum prolactin. 59th Annual Meeting of the Endocrine Society, Abstract 329.
80. Krieger, D. T., Howanitz, P. J., and Frantz, A. G. (1976): Absence of nocturnal elevation of plasma prolactin concentrations in Cushing's disease. *J. Clin. Endocrinol. Metab.*, 42:260–272.
81. Labella, F. S., Dular, R., and Vivian, S. R. (1972): Purification of bovine hypothalamic factors which inhibit (PIF) or enhance (PRF) the release of prolactin (PL) from bovine anterior pituitary *in vitro.* In: *Excerpta Medica International Congress Series 256,* p. 141. Excerpta Medica, Amsterdam.
82. Lachelin, G. C. L., Abu-Fadil, S., and Yen, S. S. C. (1977): Functional delineation of hyperprolactinemic amenorrhea. *J. Clin. Endocrinol. Metab.*, 44:1163–1174.
83. Lachelin, G. C. L., Leblanc, H., and Yen, S. S. C. (1977): The inhibitory effect of dopamine agonists on LH release in women. *J. Clin. Endocrinol. Metab.*, 44:728–732.
84. Lamberts, S. W. J., and MacLeod, R. M. (1978): Studies on the mechanism of the GABA-mediated inhibition of prolactin secretion. *Proc. Soc. Exp. Biol. Med.*, 158:10–13.
85. Lis, M., Gilardeau, C., and Chretien, M. (1973): Effect of prolactin on corticosterone production by rat adrenals. *Clin. Res.*, 21:1027.
86. MacLeod, R. M. (1976): Regulation of prolactin secretion. In: *Frontiers in Neuroendocrinology, Vol. 4,* edited by L. Martini and W. F. Ganong, pp. 169–194. Raven Press, New York.
87. MacLeod, R. M., and Lehmeyer, J. E. (1974): Studies on the mechanism of the dopamine-mediated inhibition of prolactin secretion. *Endocrinology,* 94:1077–1085.
88. Magrini, G., Ebiner, J. R., Burckhardt, P., and Felber, J. P. (1976): Study of the relationship between plasma prolactin levels and androgen metabolism in man. *J. Clin. Endocrinol. Metab.*, 43:944–947.
89. McCormick, W. F., and Halmi, N. S. (1971): Absence of chromophobe adenomas from a large series of pituitary tumors. *Arch. Pathol.*, 92:231–238.
90. McNatty, K. P., Sawers, R. S., and McNeilly, A. S. (1974): A possible role for prolactin in control of steroid secretion by the human Graafian follicle. *Nature,* 250:653–655.
91. Mortimer, C. H., Besser, G. M., McNeilly, A. S., Marshall, J. C., Harsoulis, P., Tunbridge, W. M. G., Gomez-Pan, A., and Hall, R. (1973): Luteinising hormone and follicle stimulation hormone releasing hormone test in pa-

tients with hypothalamic-pituitary-gonadal dysfunction. *Br. Med. J.,* 4: 73–77.
92. Nagulesparen, M., Ang, V., and Jenkins, J. S. (1978): Bromocriptine treatment of males with pituitary tumours, hyperprolactinemia and hypogonadism. *Clin. Endocrinol. (Oxf.),* 9:73–79.
93. Nicoll, C. S. (1974): Physiological actions of prolactin. In: *Handbook of Physiology, Vol. IV: The Pituitary Gland and its Neuroendocrine Control,* pp. 253–292. American Physiological Society, Washington, D.C.
94. Noel, G. L., Suh, H. K., and Frantz, A. G. (1974): Prolactin release during nursing and breast stimulation in post partum and non-post partum subjects. *J. Clin. Endocrinol. Metab.,* 38:413–423.
95. Orth, D. N., and Liddle, G. W. (1971): Results of therapy in 108 patients with Cushing's syndrome. *N. Engl. J. Med.,* 285:243–247.
96. Pepperell, R. J., Evans, J. H., Brown, J. B., Smith, M. A., Healy, D., and Burger, H. G. (1977): Serum prolactin levels and the value of bromocriptine in the treatment of anovulatory infertility. *Br. J. Obstet. Gynaecol.,* 84:58–66.
97. Post, K. D., Biller, B. J., Adelman, L. S., Motlitch, M. E., Wolpert, S. M., and Reichlin, S. (1979): Results of selective transsphenoidal adenomectomy in women with galactorrhea-amenorrhea. *J.A.M.A.,* 242:158–162.
98. Quigley, M. E., Judd, S. J., Gilliland, G. B., and Yen, S. S. C. (1979): Effects of a dopamine antagonist on the release of gonadotropin and prolactin in normal women and women with hyperprolactinemic anovulation. *J. Clin. Endocrinol. Metab.,* 48:718–720.
99. Reichlin, S. (1979): The prolactinoma problem. *N. Engl. J. Med.,* 300:313–315.
100. Reyes, F. I., Gomez, C., and Faiman, C. (1977): Pathological hyperprolactinemia: A five year experience. In: *Prolactin and Human Reproduction,* edited by P. G. Crosignani and C. Robyn, pp. 259–271. Academic Press, London.
101. Robyn, C., Delvoye, V., Van Exter, C., Vekemans, M., Caupriez, A., de Nayer, P., Delogne-Desnoeck, J., and L'Hermite, M. (1977): Physiological and pharmacological factors influencing prolactin secretion and their relation to human reproduction. In: *Prolactin and Human Reproduction: Proceedings of Serono Symposium,* edited by P. G. Crosignani and C. Robyn, pp. 71–96. Academic Press, New York.
102. Rolland, R., and Schellekens, L. A. (1973): A new approach to the inhibition of puerperal lactation. *J. Obstet. Gyneacol. Br. Commonwealth,* 80:945–951.
103. Roth, J., Gorden, P., and Brace, K. (1970): Efficacy of conventional pituitary irradiation in acromegaly. *N. Engl. J. Med.,* 282:1385–1391.
104. Schally, A. V., Dupont, A., Arimura, A., Takachara, J., Redding, T. W., Clemens, J., and Shaar, C. (1976): Purification of a catecholamine-rich fraction with prolactin release-inhibiting factor (PIF) activity from porcinc hypothalami. *Acta Endocrinol. (Kbh),* 82:1–14.

105. Schally, A. V., Redding, T. W., Arimura, A., Dupont, A., and Linthicum, G. L. (1977): Isolation of Gamina-amino butyric acid from pig hypothalami and demonstration of its prolactin release-inhibiting (PIF) activity *in vivo* and *in vitro. Endocrinology,* 100:681–691.
106. Schulz, K.-D., Geiger, W., del Pozo, E., and Kunzig, H. J. (1978): Pattern of sexual steroids, prolactin, and gonadotropic hormones during prolactin inhibition in normally cycling women. *Am. J. Obstet. Gynecol.,* 132:561–566.
107. Sherman, B. M., Schlechte, J., Halmi, N. S., Chapler, F. K., Harris, C. E., Duello, T. M., Van Gilder, J., and Granner, D. K. (1978): Pathogenesis of prolactin-secreting pituitary adenomas. *Lancet,* 2:1019–1021.
108. Shome, B., and Parlow, A. (1977): Human pituitary prolactin (hPRL). The entire linear amino acid sequence. *J. Clin. Endocrinol. Metab.,* 45:1112–1115.
109. Short, R. V. (1976): Definition of the problem. The evaluation of human reproduction. *Proc. R. Soc. London,* 195:3–24.
110. Swanson, H. A., and Du Boulay, G. (1975): Borderline variants of the normal pituitary fossa. *Br. J. Radiol.,* 48:366–369.
111. Taraskevich, P. S., and Douglas, W. W. (1977): Action potentials occur in cells of the normal anterior pituitary gland and are stimulated by the hypophysiotropic peptide thryrotropin releasing hormone. *Proc. Natl. Acad. Sci. U.S.A.,* 74:4064–4067.
112. Thorner, M. O. (1977): Prolactin. *Clin. Endocrinol. Metab.,* 6:201–222.
113. Thorner, M. O. (1977): Prolactin: Clinical physiology and the significance and management of hyperprolactinemia. In: *Clinical Neuroendocrinology,* edited by L. Martini and G. M. Besser, pp. 319–361. Academic Press, New York.
114. Thorner, M. O., and Besser, G. M. (1977): Hyperprolactinaemia and gonadal function: Results of bromocriptine treatment. In: *Prolactin and Human Reproduction,* edited by P. G. Crosignani and C. Robyn, pp. 285–301. Academic Press, New York.
115. Thorner, M. O., and Besser, G. M. (1978): Bromocriptine treatment of hyperprolactinemic hypogonadism. *Acta Endocrinol.* 88 (Suppl. 216):131–146.
116. Thorner, M. O., Besser, G. M., Hagen, C., and McNeilly, A. S. (1974): Long-term treatment of galactorrhoea and hypogonadism and bromocriptine. *Br. Med. J.,* 2:419–422.
117. Thorner, M. O., Besser, G. M., Jones, A., Dacie, J., and Jones, A. E. (1975): Bromocriptine therapy of female infertility—A report of 13 pregnancies. *Br. Med. J.,* 4:694–697.
118. Thorner, M. O., Edwards, C. R. W., Charlesworth, M. B., Dacie, J. E., Moult, P. J. A., Rees, L. H., Jones, A. E., and Besser, G. M. (1979): Pregnancy in patients presenting with hyperprolactinemia. *Br. Med. J.* 2:771–774.
119. Thorner, M. O., Edwards, C. R. W., Hanker, J. P., Abraham, G., and Besser, G. M. (1977): Prolactin and gonadotropin interaction in the male.

In: *The Testis in Normal and Infertile Men,* edited by P. Troen and H. Nankin, pp. 351–366. Raven Press, New York.

120. Thorner, M. O., Schran, H. F., Evans, W. S., Rogol, A. D., Morris, J. L., and MacLeod, R. M. (1980): A broad spectrum of prolactin suppression by bromocriptine in hyperprolactinemic women: A study of serum prolactin and bromocriptine levels after acute and chronic administration of bromocriptine. *J. Clin. Endocrinol. Metab. (in press).*
121. Thorner, M. O., Hackett, J., Murad, F., and MacLeod, R. M. (1980): Calcium rather than cyclic AMP as the physiological intracellular regulator of prolactin release. Submitted to *Neuroendocrinology.*
122. Tindall, G. T., McLanahan, C. S., and Christy, J. H. (1978): Transsphenoidal microsurgery for pituitary tumors associated with hyperprolactinemia. *J. Neurosurg.,* 48:849–860.
123. Utian, W. H., Begg, G., Uinik, A. I., and Paul, M. (1975): Effects of bromocriptine and dilorotrianisene on inhibition of lactation and serum prolactin. A comparative double-blind study. *Br. J. Obstet. Gynaecol.,* 82:755–759.
124. Valverde-R. C., Chietfo, V., and Reichlin, S. (1972): Prolactin-releasing factor in porcine and rat hypothalamic tissue. *Endocrinology,* 91:982–993.
125. Varga, L., Lutterbeck, P. M., Pryor, J. S., Wenner, R., and Erb, H. (1972): Suppression of puerperal lactation with an ergot alkaloid: A double-blind study. *Br. Med. J.,* 2:743–744.
126. Vermeulen, A., Suy, E., and Rubens, R. (1977): Effect of prolactin on plasma DHEA(S) levels. *J. Clin. Endocrinol. Metab.,* 44:1222–1225.
127. Vezina, J., and Sutton, T. J. (1974): Prolactin-secreting microadenomas. Roentgenologic diagnosis. *Am. J. Roentgenol.,* 120:46–54.
128. Werder, K. von, Brendel, C., Eversmann, T., Fahlbusch, R., Muller, O. A., and Rjosk, H. K. (1979): Medical therapy of hyperprolactinemia and Cushing's disease associated with pituitary adenomas. In: *Pituitary Microadenomas,* edited by G. Faglia, M. A. Giovanelli, and R. M. MacLeod. Academic Press, London *(in press).*
129. Werder, K. von, Fahlbusch, R., Landgraf, R., Pickardt, C. R., Rjosk, H. K., and Scriba, P. C. (1978): Treatment of patients with prolactinomas. *J. Endocrinol. Invest.,* 1:47–58.
130. Williams, R. A., Jacobs, H. S., Kurtz, A. B., Millar, J. G. B., Oakley, A. W., Spathis, G. S., Sulway, M. J., and Nabarro, J. D. N. (1975): The treatment of acromegaly with special reference to transsphenoidal hypophysectomy. *Q. J. Med.,* 44:79–88.
131. Yen, S. S. C. (1977): Neuroendocrine aspects of the regulation of cyclic gonadotropin release in women. In: *Clinical Neuroendocrinology,* edited by L. Martini and G. M. Besser, pp. 175–196. Academic Press, New York.
132. Yeo, T., Thorner, M. O., Jones, A., Lowry, P. J., and Besser, G. M. (1979): The effects of dopamine, bromocriptine, lergotrile, and metoclopramide on prolactin release from continuously perfused columns of isolation rat pituitary cells. *Clin. Endocrinol. (Oxf.) (in press).*

4

Bromocriptine Therapy for Acromegaly

I. INTRODUCTION

Acromegaly is characterized by excessive production of growth hormone (GH) from a pituitary tumor. It was first described in 1886 by Marie (51). Although there may be signs and symptoms resulting from local expansion of the tumor itself, the patients most frequently present with somatic problems and metabolic derangements resulting from the high circulating GH levels.

The course of acromegaly is insidious and the diagnosis is often delayed many years until complications arise that bring patients in contact with the physician. The clinical features of acromegaly are summarized in Table 1. Although some of the symptoms are relatively minor, the metabolic effects of the untreated disease lead to an increase in morbidity and mortality from cardiovascular, cerebrovascular, or respiratory complications (81). Furthermore, since the condition is insidious the patients themselves often do not realize their disability until they have been treated.

Therapy of acromegaly has two primary goals: removal or destruction of the pituitary tumor and lowering of the circulating GH levels to normal. Treatment of the tumor mass may prevent the occurrence of local symptoms such as headache and visual disturbances. The latter result from compression of the optic chiasm secondary to suprasellar extension. The development of hypopituitarism may also be prevented by resection or destruction

TABLE 1. *Common clinical features of acromegaly*

Effects of excessive GH levels:
- Excessive growth of skin and subcutaneous and soft tissues, e.g., tongue
- Skeletal overgrowth: Hands, feet
  - Skull—vault
    - —sinuses
    - —supraorbital ridges
    - —prognathism due to lower jaw growth
    - —widening of interdental spaces
  - Vertebrae—kyphosis
- Excessive sweating
- Diabetes mellitus
- Hypertension
- Heart failure
- Goiter
- Osteoarthrosis
- Nerve compression, e.g., median nerve
- Gynecomastia

Effects of associated disorders of other anterior pituitary functions:
- Gonadal dysfunction—disorders of menstruation, impotence
- Galactorrhea

Symptoms and signs of local expansion of tumor:
- Headaches
- Visual field defects

of the tumor. Restoration of serum GH levels to normal may prevent or reverse many of the associated somatic and metabolic derangements. In the past, the two major approaches to treatment have been surgery and radiotherapy.

For many years the surgical approach in treating acromegaly used a transfrontal procedure. In recent years the transsphenoidal route has been reestablished, primarily by the pioneering work of Guiot and Hardy in applying the technological advances of the image intensifier and operating microscope (26,31). The transfrontal approach is still used, either alone or in combination with the transsphenoidal approach, to treat tumors with large suprasellar extensions.

TABLE 2. *Results of surgical therapy for acromegaly*[a]

Reference	No. of evaluable patients	Success (% of patients)	Basal serum GH (ng/ml)	Comments
Transfrontal				
58	11	64	<10	Most also had external irradiation
Transsphenoidal				
32	30	53	<5	
77	56	66	<5	
		78	<5	Overall[b]
23	29	44	≤10	Surgery alone
		59	≤10	Overall[b]
33	79	77	≤10	
49	80	88	<5	During glucose tolerance test
43	16	75	≤10	
72	61	77	≤10	
78	25	92	—	Selected series
42	80	66	≤10	
	17	82	≤10	Microadenomas
	38	68	≤10	Diffuse adenomas
	25	52	≤10	Invasive adenomas

[a] Modified from Laws et al., ref. 42.
[b] With postoperative irradiation.

The various radiotherapeutic approaches include external pituitary irradiation, local implantation of radioactive yttrium into the pituitary, and more recently, heavy particle or proton beam therapy. The latter allow an extremely high dose of irradiation to be delivered to a localized site without irradiating the surrounding structures.

In Tables 2 and 3 the results of these forms of therapy are summarized. Unfortunately, destructive therapy, including both surgery and radiotherapy, may be inadequate or even ineffective in restoring GH levels to normal. In all events, external pituitary irradiation may take up to 10 years to become fully effective (19). The choice of the optimum mode of therapy is still open to debate. The incidence of hypopituitarism—pan or partial—is similar following surgery or 10 years after external pituitary irra-

TABLE 3. *Results of radiation therapy for acromegaly*

Reference	No. of evaluable patients	Success (% of patients)	Serum GH ng/ml	Comments
Conventional Radiotherapy				
60	30	23	<7.5	
61	20	45	≤10.0	
41	16	81	<7.5	
37	10	0	<10.0	
25	10	75	≤10.0	
65	17	76	<7.5	
35	10	70	≤10.0	
19	47	73	<10.0	
		81	<10.0	16 patients at
		69	<5.0	10 years
Heavy Particle Irradiation				
44	197	51	<5.0	65 patients at
		82	<10.0	5 years
Proton Beam Therapy				
38	179	53	≤5.0	22 patients at
		77	≤10.0	5 years

Modified from Laws et al., ref. 42.

diation (19). Those patients who are treated by external pituitary irradiation may continue with active disease for a number of years before the therapy is completely effective. However, recurrence has not been reported following external pituitary irradiation. The recurrence rate following surgery is unknown; Laws and colleagues (42) have reported recurrence in one patient following "successful" surgery. As in prolactinomas, the optimum results of transsphenoidal surgery have been reported in those patients with well circumscribed tumors, particularly microadenomas. The conclusions of Eastman et al. (19) perhaps summarize the problem most succinctly: ". . . conventional supervoltage irradiation, heavy particle irradiation, (possibly proton beam irradiation), and transsphenoidal microsurgery ultimately all achieve the same fall in plasma GH levels. The treatment modalities differ, however, with regard to side effects, and in the speed with which the fall in GH levels is achieved."

Apart from the cosmetic and practical difficulties associated with their coarse features, acromegalic patients are often severely disabled by their symptoms of excessive sweating, headaches, and impotence; they also are unable to perform fine and delicate manual functions due to thickening of soft tissues. Furthermore, lack of restoration of the normal hormonal balance is presumably still associated with the enhanced morbidity and mortality of the condition. For these reasons there has been a long search for an effective medical treatment to supplement surgery and/or radiotherapy directed at the pituitary tumor. Estrogens, chlorpromazine, and medroxyprogesterone acetate have each been proclaimed as effective but have not stood up to clinical trial (20). The discovery of somatostatin and its efficacy in lowering GH in acromegalics (1,2,29) raised the hope that this would be an effective therapy. Somatostatin, however, has widespread effects of inhibition of the release of many other hormones, including insulin, glucagon, renin, gastrin, vasoactive intestinal peptide, gastric inhibitory peptide, and motilin. These untoward effects, coupled with its extreme brevity of action and the need for parenteral administration, have made the use of somatostatin impractical for therapy of acromegaly, although it remains a fascinating research tool.

II. CONTROL OF GROWTH HORMONE SECRETION

The anterior pituitary hormones are synthesized and released under the control of the hypothalamus, which secretes regulatory hormones at the median eminence into portal capillaries. The portal capillaries then transport the regulatory hormones to the anterior pituitary, where they exert their specific effects. The hypothalamic regulatory hormones are synthesized in peptidergic neurons in the hypothalamus and their release is controlled by neurotransmitters in the hypothalamus, including the catecholamines, serotonin, histamine, substance P, and probably endogenous opiate agonists (e.g., endorphins and/or enkephalins). Growth hormone secretion is controlled by two hypothalamic regulatory hormones, growth hormone releasing factor (GRF, which has yet to be characterized) and GH release inhibiting hormone (somatostatin). Growth hormone produces some or all of its biological effects through somatomedin, a peptide(s) produced in the liver (16). The physiological factors that control growth hormone secretion, including those responsible for feedback on its release, are not established; this subject has recently been extensively reviewed (15,52,59).

A fundamental and as yet unresolved question is whether acromegaly is primarily a pituitary or hypothalamic disease. However, the apparent cure of many patients by selective adenoma removal lends support to the view that acromegaly is primarily, at least in certain patients, a pituitary disease.

The knowledge that pituitary hormones, including GH, are under hypothalamic regulatory hormone control, and that these in turn are under neurotransmitter control, has led several groups to investigate the role of neurotransmitters on growth hormone release in normal subjects and in acromegalics.

TABLE 4. *Effects of drugs that stimulate (agonist) or block (antagonist) adrenoreceptors on growth hormone release in man*

Receptor	Normal subjects		Acromegalic subjects	
	Agonist	Antagonist	Agonist	Antagonist
α Adreno receptor	↑ (40)	↓ (52)	—	↓ (13,14,47)
β Receptor	—	↑ (4,52)	—	—
Dopamine receptor	↑ (5,71)	↓ (66)	↓ (7,9–11, 45, 62,70,71)	→ (17,47) or ↓ (39,63)
Serotonin receptor	→ (54,80) or ?↑ (67)	—	→ (55)	→ (79)

Note: Arrows indicate stimulation, inhibition, or no change in growth hormone secretion. Reference numbers in parentheses.

The effects of stimulation and blockade of various receptors on GH secretion in normal and acromegalic subjects are shown in Table 4. However, although the compounds used were chosen for their specificity, no drug is a pure agonist or antagonist, and they often interfere with a variety of other receptors (56).

III. BROMOCRIPTINE THERAPY FOR ACROMEGALY

A. Rationale for Bromocriptine Therapy

In normal subjects an acute dose of levodopa causes stimulation of GH. The observation by Liuzzi and colleagues (46) that GH falls in some acromegalics following levodopa led to a search for a drug that would produce this effect during chronic therapy; levodopa itself was ineffective during chronic therapy, probably because of its short duration of action (9). The same group, therefore, investigated the role of bromocriptine, a long-acting dopamine agonist, and found a single oral 2.5 mg dose to be effective in lowering GH levels for several hours in a group of acromegalic patients (45). The Italian group, the group at St. Bartholomew's Hospital, London, the group in Newcastle upon Tyne, as well as several others, then evaluated the efficacy of long-term bromocriptine treatment in acromegaly (10,62,70). The results of these separate studies have been similar, and although GH levels are rarely restored to normal, the clinical and metabolic responses have been excellent. These will be discussed in detail below.

The mechanism by which dopamine agonists lower GH levels in acromegaly is still not clear. It is known that GH-secreting cells in patients with acromegaly remain under some hypothalamic control, since GH levels rise during hypoglycemia, and in many patients there is a paradoxical rise after an oral glucose load (in contrast to normal subjects, in whom GH levels are suppressed following a glucose load). Besser and colleagues (2) suggested that acromegaly may result from somatostatin deficiency, since the paradoxical rise of growth hormone after an oral glucose load can be abolished by a somatostatin infusion.

However, irrespective of whether the primary abnormality is hypothalamic or pituitary, some hypothalamic influence over growth hormone secretion is preserved in acromegaly. Thus, dopamine agonists may exert their effects either at the hypothalamic or the pituitary level. If they act on the hypothalamus their mode of action may be either to inhibit GRF secretion or to stimulate somatostatin secretion or both. In normal subjects the net effect of acute dopamine receptor stimulation is GH release, and this is thought to be a hypothalamic effect (5,71,73). In contrast, in acromegaly, dopamine agonists probably act at the pituitary level. Drugs that act at the hypothalamic level, as pointed out by Liuzzi and colleagues (47), are ineffective in lowering GH levels in acromegalics—for example, amphetamine, which acts to release catecholamines, including dopamine. Furthermore, infusions of lower doses of dopamine than are necessary to release GH in normal subjects are effective in lowering GH levels in acromegalics (73). Since dopamine is poorly transported across the blood-brain barrier, these data suggest the drug acts either at the median eminence, which is outside the blood-brain barrier, or at the pituitary level. Release of GH from fragments of human GH-secreting pituitary tumors can be inhibited by the dopamine agonist, bromocriptine, *in vitro* (36,53). Furthermore, these cells can be stimulated to secrete growth hormone by thyrotropin-releasing hormone (36). These data are compatible with the view that such tumors may represent a dedifferentiation of somato-mammotropic cells to their more primitive lactotrope characteristics (47,48). This concept is supported by data that suggest prolactin and GH can be secreted by the same cells (27).

This conclusion is supported by the report of one acromegalic patient who had a paradoxical response to levodopa and a GH response to TRH before removal of his tumor. Following selective adenectomy the normal hormonal responses were restored, suggesting that no permanent derangement of control of GH secretion existed in the hypothalamus or in the remainder of the pituitary (34). It has been suggested that there is concordance between those patients who responded to TRH with an increase in GH release and those who responded to bromocriptine with a fall, but Wass and colleagues found that although this was generally true, there were exceptions *(see page 114)*. Under different pathological conditions, including renal (24) and hepatic (57) failure, anorexia nervosa (50) and depression, and hypothyroidism (30), TRH results in a rise in GH levels. Furthermore, in some patients with acromegaly, GnRH leads to a rise in GH; however, there is no homogeneity of responses to TRH and GnRH in these patients (21,22). The significance of these anomolous responses is still not clear.

Dopamine (73), as well as other dopamine agonists, including levodopa (46), apomorphine (47), piribedil (7), methergoline (11), lergotrile (71), and lisuride (47), are effective in lowering GH levels; the ergot derivatives methergoline, lergotrile, and lisuride have been used in chronic therapy for acromegaly. However, the greatest experience has been with bromocriptine, and the other ergot drugs do not appear to offer any great advantages. For that reason all the discussion will be limited to experience with bromocriptine.

B. Results of Bromocriptine Therapy (Table 5)

Bromocriptine appears to be the first effective medical therapy for acromegaly. The results of therapy should be considered not only in terms of the fall in GH levels, but also in terms of clinical and metabolic responses.

1. Growth Hormone Suppression

The results of some of the largest series are summarized in Table 5. Although the results vary, the largest single series is that from St. Bartholomew's Hospital in London, where more than 100 patients have now been treated (3). The criteria used for a significant fall in GH levels vary with each group. The Italian group has been the most conservative and requires a fall of at least 50% to represent a significant decline, whereas the

TABLE 5. *Results of bromocriptine therapy for acromegaly*

Reference	No. of patients	Dose (mg/day)	Duration (months)	Percentage with fall in GH levels			Percentage with clinical improvement
				Total	<10	<5 ng/ml	
10	12	10	1–12	58	50	33	58
62	21	10–60	6–10	90	57	19	100
76	10	20–60[a]	?	30	—	20	60
18	5	20	3	40	—	—	40
64	22	7.5–50	3–22	77	68	59	77
8	12	7.5–30	6	92	58	33	25
6	19	10–40	?	79	37	—	73
3	101	10–60	9–60	77	—	19	94
68	5	7.5–15	6	60	—	—	60

[a] Given on a twice daily regimen.

London group considers a fall of greater than 7 ng/ml in the mean serum GH levels through the day to be significant. The London results will be considered in greatest detail, since one of the authors (M.O.T.) was directly involved in the study. This study has now been in progress for 5 years.

The initial report by Liuzzi and colleagues (45) on the effects of acute administration of a single 2.5 mg dose of bromocriptine to acromegalics showed that GH levels could be lowered for several hours. Early studies clearly indicated that the duration of suppression of GH after 2.5 mg of bromocriptine was shorter than for suppression of prolactin. Thus, the London group increased the dose and frequency of administration from 2.5 mg every 12 hr to 5 mg every 6 hr, which resulted in prolonged suppression of GH levels (Fig. 1).

The optimal dose of bromocriptine in acromegaly has not been established; each patient appears to have his own optimal dose. Brooks and colleagues (6) examined the effects of four different

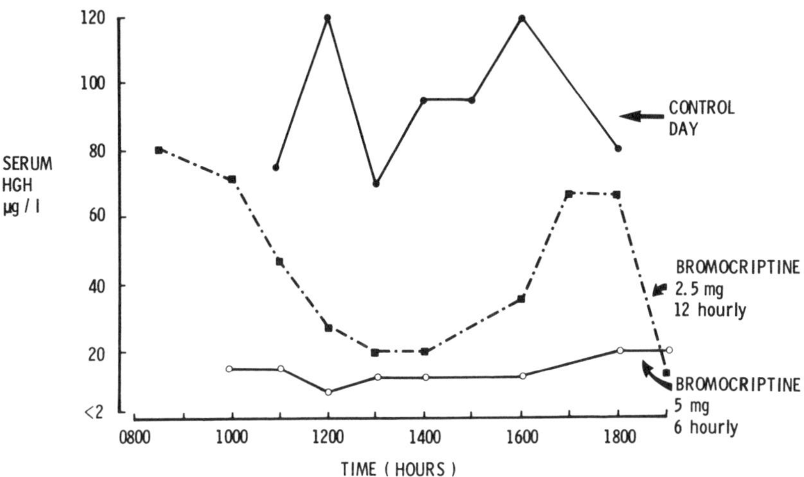

FIG. 1. Serum growth hormone levels during the day in an acromegalic female before treatment (control day), on bromocriptine 2.5 mg every 12 hr, and on bromocriptine 5 mg every 6 hr. (Reproduced with permission from Thorner et al., ref. 70.)

doses—10, 20, 30, and 40 mg/day—in 19 acromegalic patients. They found the optimal dose for suppression of GH levels to be 20 mg/day in four divided doses. However, serum GH levels only fell in two patients on doses of 30 and 40 mg/day. In contrast, Wass and associates (75) progressively increased the dose above 20 mg/day in 21 patients, and further lowering of mean GH levels through the day was observed in 12 patients; however, increasing the dose above that at which the maximal lowering of GH levels was seen did not have any additional effect (3,75).

It is thus not surprising that recommendations for dosages have varied from 10 to 60 mg/day (10,62,70,75). However, the total dose should be given in four divided doses throughout the day. In Fig. 2 the mean serum GH levels in 101 acromegalics before and during bromocriptine therapy is shown. The duration of treatment was from 9 to 60 months (3).

In the results of long-term therapy reported by Wass and colleagues (75), the 58 "responsive" patients (whose GH levels fell by greater than 7 ng/ml), 15 (26%) had levels on treatment of equal to or less than 5 ng/ml, 10 (17%) had levels of 6 to 10 ng/ml, 17 (29%) had levels of 11 to 20 ng/ml, and only 16 (28%) had levels above 20 ng/ml. Thus, GH levels were maintained below 10 ng/ml through the day in 43%, and only 28% of "responsive" patients had GH levels above 20 ng/ml. Furthermore, in only 3 of the 58 patients was the initial reduction in GH not maintained with chronic treatment; in none of the 3 did GH reach pretreatment levels. However, it must be stressed that mean serum GH levels in normal subjects are less than 5 ng/ml and therefore, serum GH levels are, in general, not restored to normal by bromocriptine therapy.

Acromegalic patients have abnormal responses to TRH, LHRH, and oral glucose loading. In the patients described by Wass and colleagues (75), the responses to TRH and glucose were tested before and during bromocriptine therapy. Twenty-nine of 35 acromegalic patients showed a rise in GH levels of greater than 10 ng/ml after TRH prior to bromocriptine therapy. Of those 29, 11 were tested again during treatment with bromo-

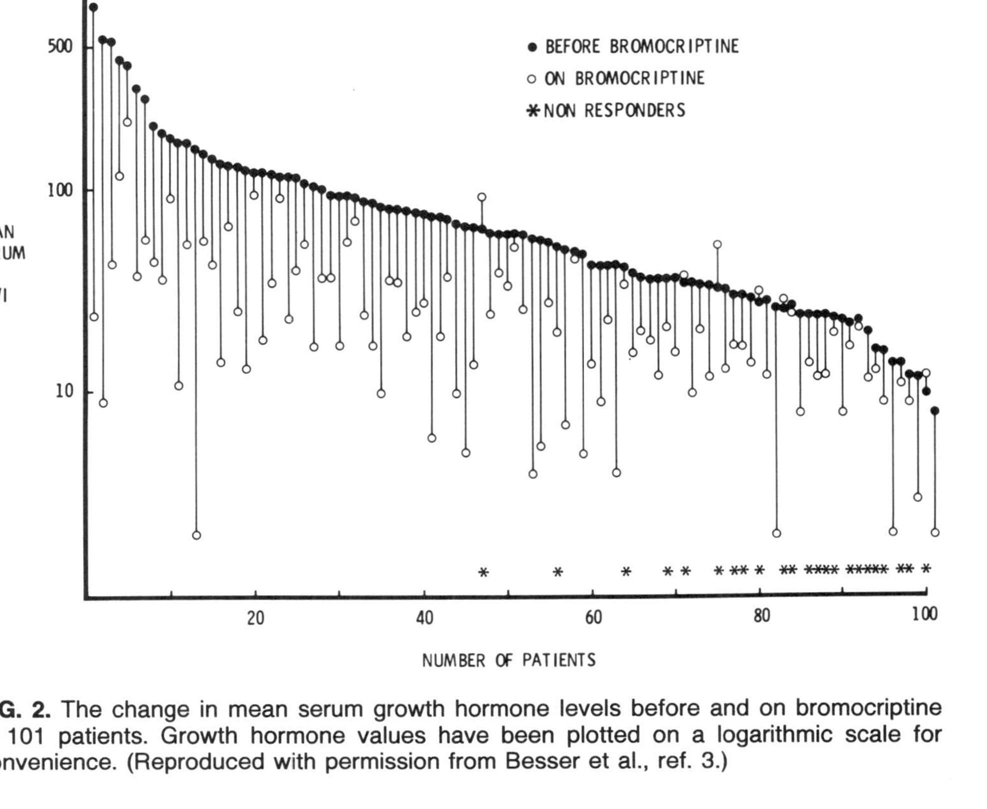

FIG. 2. The change in mean serum growth hormone levels before and on bromocriptine in 101 patients. Growth hormone values have been plotted on a logarithmic scale for convenience. (Reproduced with permission from Besser et al., ref. 3.)

criptine. The GH response to TRH was abolished in 7. Two patients, whose GH levels did not rise in response to TRH before therapy, showed a good response to chronic bromocriptine therapy, whereas 3 patients in whom there was a clear rise in growth hormone to TRH did not respond to therapy.

Prior to treatment, 22 patients demonstrated a paradoxical rise in GH following an oral glucose load. This response was abolished in 15 patients after 12 months on bromocriptine therapy.

2. Metabolic Response

Associated with the reduction of GH levels in acromegalics treated with bromocriptine, there were objective metabolic changes, including a reduction in collagen turnover, as measured by urinary hydroxyproline excretion (70), and improvement in glucose tolerance (3,10,70,75). Of the 73 patients reported by Wass and colleagues, 32% had chemical diabetes mellitus before treatment and 87% of these demonstrated improvement in glucose tolerance. During chronic treatment, glucose tolerance eventually became normal in 65%.

At least some of the GH-induced metabolic effects are mediated through the somatomedins (12,28,69). However, documentation of changes in serum somatomedin concentrations has appeared in only one study (76). However, in this study the numbers were small and it is difficult to draw any conclusions from it.

3. Clinical Response

Ninety-seven percent of patients reported by Wass and colleagues (75) noted some symptomatic improvements: cessation or reduction of excessive sweating occurred in 60 of 63 patients with this symptom, improvement of greasiness and thickness of skin occurred in 42, facial features improved in 26, 56 patients noticed changes in hand and finger sizes, and 31 patients noted a decrease in their foot size. Other changes noted by the patients included improvement in libido and sexual performance in 17 of the men; 12, however, were hyperprolactinemic before treatment. Another 15 patients noted improvement in general well being. Objective evaluation revealed a reduction in ring size in 30 of 34 patients measured through 1 year of therapy (Figure 3). There was improvement in hypertension in 8 of 29 patients and relief of headache in 15 of 20. Visual fields improved in 2 patients within 3 months of therapy (1 of whom had also been treated by external irradiation). There was no change in the skull X-ray appearances in 45 patients treated for 1 year. However, subsequent evidence of tumor shrinkage was observed in 20% of acromegalic patients, but the majority of these patients had also undergone external pituitary irradiation (74).

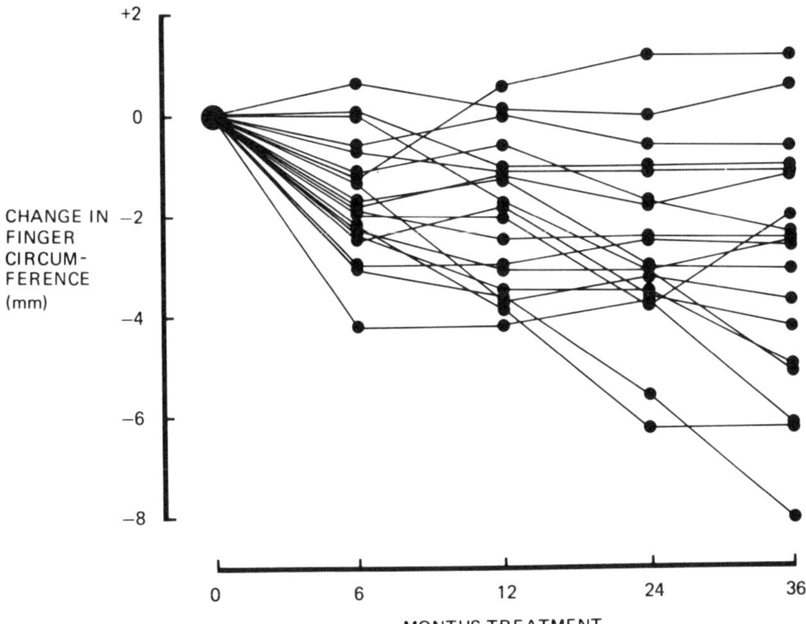

FIG. 3. The change in finger circumference in 19 patients during bromocriptine treatment (given for 36 months). (Reproduced with permission from Besser et al., ref. 3.)

4. Withdrawal of Bromocriptine

The effects of withdrawal of bromocriptine therapy in acromegalic patients was observed over a 2-month period, following 12 months of therapy. A rise in GH levels, usually to lower levels than those seen before therapy, was seen and this elevation was associated with worsening of glucose tolerance in the diabetic patients. This group experienced a return of the symptoms of acromegaly, including excessive sweating, headaches, and decrease in potency and well being.

5. Tumor Growth

The effects of bromocriptine and other dopamine agonists on tumor growth will be discussed in Chapter 7. There is evidence, based on improvement in visual fields, reduction in tumor size as documented by CAT scans, and in experimental animal models, that dopamine agonists can reduce tumor growth (particularly prolactin-secreting tumors) in certain instances. The data, however, are preliminary. After 1 to 5 years of bromocriptine therapy associated with external pituitary irradiation, approximately 20% of tumors in acromegalic or hyperprolactinemic patients show evidence of regression (3,74,75).

6. Bromocriptine Administration

To avoid the initial side effects of dopamine agonist therapy, it is advisable to begin therapy with a small dose and gradually increase it. Thus, 2.5 mg bromocriptine is given orally with food on retiring and every 3 days a further dose is administered until the patient is taking 2.5 mg four times daily with food. Depending on the dosage schedule adopted by the physician, either this dose is maintained or it is increased in the same manner to 5 mg four times daily. The author recommends that 2.5 mg four times daily be maintained for 3 months, followed by evaluation of the clinical response. If the patient exhibits an acceptable response, the dose should be maintained. If, however, there has been an inadequate response, the dose is increased until an acceptable response is seen or a maximum dose of 60 mg/day is achieved.

IV. CONCLUSIONS

Bromocriptine is effective and useful in reversing many of the clinical and metabolic effects of excessive GH secretion seen in acromegaly. However, it does not restore GH levels to normal in the majority of patients.

Acromegaly is almost always associated with a pituitary tumor. Surgical or radiotherapeutic approaches are the first line of treatment and should be used unless contraindicated. If a patient is left with active acromegaly following primary therapy directed at the pituitary tumor, then medical treatment with bromocriptine is indicated. It is frequently effective and appears to be safe. Following its withdrawal, patients often revert to their pretreatment state. Adverse effects of therapy occur; they are often minimal and do not prevent continuation of therapy *(see Chapter 6)*. Therapy is expensive; however, physicians should not minimize the symptoms and disability caused by acromegaly. Hopefully, medical therapy will help prevent the complications associated with acromegaly when primary treatment directed at the pituitary has not been fully effective or has not achieved its full potential, since, for example, external pituitary irradiation may take up to 10 years to produce its maximal effects.

REFERENCES

1. Besser, G. M., Mortimer, C. H., Carr, D., Schally, A. V., Coy, D. H. Evered, D. C., Kastin, A. J., Tunbridge, W. M. G., Thorner, M. O., and Hall, R. (1974): Growth hormone-release inhibiting hormone in acromegaly. *Br. Med. J.,* 1:352 355.
2. Besser, G. M., Mortimer, C. H., McNeilly, A. S., Thorner, M. O., Batistoni, G. A., Bloom, S. R., Kastrup, K. W., Hansen, K. F., Hall, R., Coy, D. H., Kastin, A. J., and Schally, A. V. (1974): Long-term infusions of growth hormone-release inhibiting hormone in acromegaly: Effects on pituitary and pancreatic hormones. *Br. Med. J.,* 4:622–627.

3. Besser, G. M., Wass, J. A. H., and Thorner, M. O. (1979): Bromocriptine treatment of acromegaly. In: *Ergot Compounds and Brain Function—Neuroendocrine and Neuropsychiatric Aspects,* edited by G. Goldstein, A. Lieberman, D. B. Calne, and M. Thorner. Raven Press, New York *(in press).*
4. Blackard, W. G., and Heidingsfelder, S. A. (1968): Adrenergic receptor control mechanism for growth hormone secretion. *J. Clin. Invest.,* 47:1407–1414.
5. Boyd, A. E., Lebovitz, H. E., and Pfeiffer (1970): Stimulation of growth hormone secretion by L-dopa. *N. Engl. J. Med.,* 283:1425–1429.
6. Brooks, A. P., Stephen, P. J., Nairn, I. M., and Strong, J. A. (1979): Bromocriptine and acromegaly: Therapeutic implications. *J. R. Soc. Med.,* 72:562–564.
7. Camanni, F., Massara, F., Fassio, U., Molinatti, G. M., and Muller, E. E. (1975): Effect of five dopaminergic drugs on plasma growth hormone levels in acromegalic subjects. *Neuroendocrinology,* 19:227–240.
8. Cassar, J., Mashiter, K., and Joplin, G. F. (1977): Bromocriptine treatment of acromegaly. *Metabolism,* 26:539–547.
9. Chiodini, P. G., Liuzzi, A., Botalla, L., Cremascoli, G., and Silvestrini, F. (1974): Inhibitory effect of dopaminergic stimulation on GH release in acromegaly. *J. Clin. Endocrinol. Metab.,* 38:200–206.
10. Chiodini, P. G., Liuzzi, A., Botalla, L., Oppizzi, G., Muller, E. E., and Silvestrini, F. (1975): Stable reduction of plasma growth hormone (hGH) levels during chronic administration of 2-Br-α-ergocryptine (CB-154) in acromegalic patients. *J. Clin. Endocrinol. Metab.,* 40:705–708.
11. Chiodini, P. G., Liuzzi, A., Muller, E. E., Botalla, L., Cremascoli, G., Oppizzi, G., Verde, G., and Silvestrini, F. (1976): Inhibitory effect of an ergoline derivative, methergoline, on growth hormone and prolactin levels in acromegalic patients. *J. Clin. Endocrinol. Metab.,* 43:356–363.
12. Chochinov, R. H., and Daughaday, W. H. (1976): Current concepts of somatomedin and other biologically related growth factors. *Diabetes,* 25:997–1004.
13. Cryer, P. E., and Daughaday, W. H. (1974): Adrenergic modulation of growth hormone secretion in acromegaly: Suppression during phentolamine and phentolamine-isoproterenol administration. *J. Clin. Endocrinol. Metab.,* 39:658–663.
14. Cryer, P. E., and Daughaday, W. H. (1977): Adrenergic modulation of growth hormone secretion in acromegaly: Alpha- and beta-adrenergic blockade produce qualitatively normal responses but no effect on L-dopa suppression. *J. Clin. Endocrinol. Metab.,* 44:977–999.
15. Cryer, P. E., and Daughaday, W. H. (1977): Growth hormone. In: *Clinical Neuroendocrinology,* edited by L. Martini and G. M. Besser, pp. 243–277. Academic Press, New York.
16. Daughaday, W. H. (1978): Hormonal regulation of growth by somatomedin and other tissue growth factors. *Clin. Endocrinol. Metabol.,* 6:117–135.
17. Dimond, R. C., Brammer, S. R., Atkinson, R. L., Jr., Howard, W. J., and Earl, J. M. (1973): Chlorpromazine treatment and growth hormone

secretory responses in acromegaly. *J. Clin. Endocrinol. Metab.,* 36:1189–1195.

18. Dunn, P. J., Donald, R. A., and Espiner, E. A. (1977): Bromocriptine suppression of plasma growth hormone in acromegaly. *Clin. Endocrinol. (Oxf.),* 7:273–281.
19. Eastman, R. C., Gorden, P., and Roth, J. (1979): Conventional supervoltage irradiation is an effective treatment for acromegaly. *J. Clin. Endocrinol. Metab.,* 48:931–940.
20. Eastman, R. C., and Roth, J. (1978): Acromegaly. In: *Clinical Pharmacology: Basic Principals in Therapeutics,* edited by K. L. Melmon and H. F. Morelli, pp. 560–562. Macmillan, London.
21. Faglia, G., Beck-Peccoz, P., Ferrari, C., Travaglini, P., Ambrosi, B., and Spada, A. (1973): Plasma growth hormone response to thyrotropin-releasing hormone in patients with active acromegaly. *J. Clin. Endocrinol. Metab.,* 36:1259–1262.
22. Faglia, G., Beck-Peccoz, P., Travaglini, P., Paracchi, A., Spada, A., and Levin, A. (1973): Elevations in plasma growth hormone concentration after luteinizing hormone-releasing hormone (LRH) in patients with active acromegaly. *J. Clin. Endocrinol. Metab.,* 37:338–340.
23. Giovanelli, M. A., Motti, E. D. F., and Paracchi, A. (1976): Treatment of acromegaly by transsphenoidal microsurgery. *J. Neurosurg.,* 44:677–686.
24. Gonzalez-Barcena, D., Kastin, A. J., Schlach, D. S., Torres-Zamora, M., Perez-Paten, E., Kato, E., and Schally, A. V. (1973): Response to thyrotropin-releasing hormone in patients with renal failure and after insulin in normal men. *J. Clin. Endocrinol. Metab.,* 36:117–120.
25. Gorden, P., and Roth, J. (1973): The treatment of acromegaly by conventional pituitary irradiation. In: *Diagnosis and Treatment of Pituitary Tumors,* edited by P. O. Kohler and G. T. Ross, pp. 230–233. Excerpta Medica International Congress Series No. 303, Amsterdam.
26. Guiot, G., Rougerie, J., and Brion, S. (1958): L'utilization des amplificateurs de brilliance en neuroradiologie et dans la chirurgie stereotaxique. *Ann. Chir.,* 34:689–695.
27. Guyda, H., Robert, F., Colle, E., and Hardy, J. (1973): Histologic, ultrastructural, and hormonal characterisation of a pituitary tumor secreting both hGH and prolactin. *J. Clin. Endocrinol. Metab.,* 36:531–547.
28. Hall, K., Takano, K., and Fryklund, L. (1974): Radioreceptor assay for somatomedin A. *J. Clin. Endocrinol. Metab.,* 39:973–976.
29. Hall, R., Besser, G. M., Schally, A. V., Coy, D. H., Evered, D. C., Goldie, D. J., Kastin, A. J., McNeilly, A. S., Mortimer, C. H., Phenekos, C., Tunbridge, W. M. G., and Weightman, D. R. (1973): Actions of growth hormone-release inhibiting hormone in healthy men and in acromegaly. *Lancet,* 2:581–584.
30. Hamada, N., Voi, K., Nishizawa, Y., Okamoto, T., Hasegawa, K., Morii, H., and Wada, M. (1976): Increase in serum GH concentration following TRH injection in patients with primary hypothyroidism. *Endocrinol. Jpn.,* 23:5–10.

31. Hardy, J. (1973): Transsphenoidal surgery of hypersecreting pituitary tumors. In: *Diagnosis and Treatment of Pituitary Tumours,* edited by P. O. Kohler and G. T. Ross, pp. 179–194. Excerpta Medica International Congress Series, No. 303, Amsterdam.
32. Hardy, J., Robert, F., Somma, M., and Vezina, J. L. (1973): Acromégalie-gigantisme traitment chirurgical par exérèse transphénoidale de l'adénome hypophysaire. *Neurochirurgie,* 19(Suppl. 2):1–178.
33. Hardy, J., Somma, M., and Vezina, J. L. (1976): Treatment of acromegaly: Radiation or surgery? In: *Current Controversies in Neurosurgery,* edited by T. P. Morley, pp. 377–391. W. B. Saunders, Philadelphia.
34. Hoyte, K. M., and Martin, J. B. (1975): Recovery from paradoxical growth hormone responses in acromegaly after transsphenoidal selective adenectomy. *J. Clin. Endocrinol. Metab.,* 41:656–659.
35. Hunter, W. M., Gillingham, F. J., Harris, P., Kanis, J. A., McGurr, F. M., McLelland, J., and Strong, J. A. (1974): Serial assays of plasma growth hormone in treated and untreated acromegaly. *J. Endocrinol.,* 63:21–34.
36. Ishibashi, M., and Yamaji, T. (1978): Effect of thyrotropin releasing hormone and bromoergocriptine on growth hormone and prolactin secretion in perfused pituitary adenoma tissues of acromegaly. *J. Clin. Endocrinol. Metab.,* 47:1251–1256.
37. Jenkins, J. S., Ash, S., and Bloom, H. J. G. (1972): Endocrine function after external irradiation in patients with secreting and non-secreting pituitary tumors. *Q. J. Med.,* 41:57–69.
38. Kjellberg, R. N., and Kliman, B. (1973): A system for therapy of pituitary tumors. In: *Diagnosis and Treatment of Pituitary Tumors,* edited by P. O. Kohler and G. T. Ross, pp. 234–252. Excerpta Medica International Congress Series No. 303, Amsterdam.
39. Kolodny, H. D., Sherman, L. S., Singh, A., Kim, S., and Benjamin, F. (1971): Acromegaly treated with chlorpromazine, *N. Engl. J. Med.,* 284:819–822.
40. Lal, S., Tolis, G., Martin, J. B., Brown, G. M., and Guyda, H. (1975): Effects of clonidine on growth hormone, prolactin, luteinizing hormone, follicle-stimulating hormone and thyroid-stimulating hormone in serum of normal men. *J. Clin. Endocrinol. Metab.,* 41:703–708.
41. Lawrence, A. M., Pinsky, S. M., and Goldfine, I. D. (1971): Conventional radiation therapy in acromegaly: A review and reassessment. *Arch. Intern. Med.,* 128:369–377.
42. Laws, E. R., Jr., Piepgras, D. G., Randall, R. V., and Abboud, C. F. (1979): Neurosurgical management of acromegaly: Results in 82 patients treated between 1972 and 1977. *J. Neurosurg.,* 50:454–461.
43. Leavans, M. E., Samaan, N. A., and Jesse, R. H., Jr. (1977): Clinical and endocrinological evaluation of 16 acromegalic patients treated by transsphenoidal surgery. *J. Neurosurg.,* 47:853–860.
44. Linfoot, J. A., Nakagawa, J. S., Wiedemann, E., Lyman, J., Chong, C., Garcia, J., and Lawrence, J. H.: Heavy particle therapy: Pituitary tumors. Quoted in ref. 19.

45. Liuzzi, A., Chiodini, P. G., Botalla, L., Cremascoli, G., Muller, E. E., and Silvestrini, F. (1974): Decreased plasma growth hormone (GH) levels in acromegalics following CB 154 (2-Br-α-ergocryptine) administration. *J. Clin. Endocrinol. Metab.,* 38:910–912.
46. Liuzzi, A., Chiodini, P. G., Botalla, L., Cremascoli, G., and Silvestrini, F. (1972): Inhibitory effect of L-dopa on GH release in acromegalic patients. *J. Clin. Endocrinol. Metab.,* 35:941–943.
47. Liuzzi, A., Chiodini, P. G., Silvestrini, F., Cozzi, R., Opizzi, G., Botalla, L., and Verde, G. (1979): Effects of neuroactive drugs on growth hormone and prolactin secretion in acromegaly. In: *Pituitary Microadenomas,* edited by G. Faglia, M. A. Giovanelli, and R. M. MacLeod. Academic Press, London *(in press).*
48. Liuzzi, A., Panerai, A. E., Chiodini, P. G., Secchi, C., Cocchi, D., Botalla, L., Silvestrini, F., and Muller, E. E. (1975): Neuroendocrine control of growth hormone secretion: Experimental and clinical studies. In: *Growth Hormone and Related Peptides,* edited by E. Pecile and E. E. Muller, pp. 236–251. Excerpta Medica, Amsterdam.
49. Lüdecke, D., Kantzky, R., and Saeger, W. (1976): Selective removal of hypersecreting pituitary adenomas? An analysis of endocrine function, operative and microscopical findings in 101 cases. *Acta Neurochir. (Wein),* 35:27–42.
50. Maeda, K., Kato, Y., Oligo, S., Chihara, K., Yoshimoto, Y., Yamaguchi, N., Kuromaru, S., and Imura, H. (1975): Growth hormone and prolactin release after injection of thyrotropin-releasing hormone in patients with depression. *J. Clin. Endocrinol. Metab.,* 40:501–505.
51. Marie, P. (1886): Sur deux cas d'acromegalie. *Rev. Med.,* 6:297.
52. Martin, J. B. (1976): Brain regulation of growth hormone secretion. In: *Frontiers in Neuroendocrinology, Vol. 4,* edited by L. Martini and W. F. Ganong, pp. 129–168. Raven Press, New York.
53. Mashiter, K., Adams, E., Beard, M., and Holley, A. (1977): Bromocriptine inhibits prolactin and growth hormone release by human pituitary tumours in culture. *Lancet,* 2:197–198.
54. Muller, E. E., Brambilla, F., Cavagnini, F., Paracchi, P., and Panerai, A. (1974): Slight effect on L-tryptophan on growth hormone release in normal human subjects. *J. Clin. Endocrinol. Metab.,* 39:1–5.
55. Oppizzi, G., Cremascoli, G., De Stefano, L., Colussi, G., Verde, G., Liuzzi, A., Chiodini, P. G., and Botalla, L. (1876): Serotonina, dopamina e neuroregoluzione dell 'ormone somatotrope. Atti Del XVI Congresso Società Italiana di Endocrinologi, Abstract 31.
56. Oppizzi, G., Verde, G., De Stefano, L., Cozzi, R., Botalla, L., Liuzzi, A., and Chiodini, P. G. (1977): Evidence for a dopaminergic activity of methysergide in humans. *Clin. Endocrinol. (Oxf.),* 7:267–272.
57. Panerai, A. E., Salerno, F., Manneschi, M., Cocchi, D., and Muller, E. E. (1977): Growth hormone and prolactin responses to thyrotropin-releasing hormone in patients with severe liver disease. *J. Clin. Endocrinol. Metab.,* 45:134–140.

58. Ray, B. S., Horwith, M., and Mautalen, C. (1968): Surgical hypophysectomy as a treatment for acromegaly. In: *Clinical Endocrinology, Vol. 2,* edited by E. B. Astwood and C. E. Cassidy, pp. 93–102. Grue and Stratton, New York.
59. Reichlin, S. (1974): Regulation of somatotrophic hormone secretion. In: *Handbook of Physiology, Vol. IV, Sect 7: Endocrinology: The Pituitary and its Neuroendocrine Control,* pp. 405–447. American Physiological Society, Washington, D.C.
60. Roth, J., Glick, S. M., Cantrecasas, P., and Hollander, C. S. (1967): Acromegaly and other disorders of growth hormone secretion. Combined clinical staff conference at the National Institutes of Health. *Ann. Intern. Med.,* 66:760–788.
61. Roth, J., Gorden, P., and Brace, K. (1970). Efficacy of conventional pituitary irradiation in acromegaly. *N. Engl. J. Med.,* 282:1385–1391.
62. Sachdev, Y., Gomez-Pan, A., Tunbridge, W. M. G., Dunns, A., Weightman, D. R., Hall, R., and Goolamali, S. K. (1975): Bromocriptine therapy in acromegaly. *Lancet,* 2:1164–1168.
63. Schaison, G., Croisner, J. C., Nathan, C., and Dreyfus, G. (1974): Essai de traitment de l'acromegalie par le sulpiride. *Ann. Endocrinol.,* 35:103–110.
64. Schwinn, G., Dirks, H., McIntosh, C., and Köbberling, J. (1977): Metabolic and clinical studies in patients with acromegaly treated with bromocriptine over 22 months. *Eur. J. Clin. Invest.,* 7:101–107.
65. Sheline, G. E. (1973): Treatment of chromophobe adenomas of the pituitary gland and acromegaly. In: *Diagnosis and Treatment of Pituitary Tumors,* edited by P. O. Kohler and G. T. Ross, pp. 230–233. Excerpta Medica International Congress Series No. 303, Amsterdam.
66. Sherman, L., Kim, S., and Benjamin, F. (1971): Effect of chlorpromazine on serum growth hormone concentration in man. *N. Engl. J. Med.,* 284:72–74.
67. Smythe, G. A. (1977): Role of serotonin and dopamine in hypothalamic-pituitary function. *Clin. Endocrinol. (Oxf.),* 7:325–341.
68. Spark, R. F., and Dickstein, G. (1979): Bromocriptine and endocrine disorders. *Ann. Intern. Med.,* 90:949–956.
69. Takano, K., Hall, K., Ritzen, M., Iselius, L., and Sievertsson, H. (1976): Somatomedin A in human serum, determined by radioreceptor assay. *Acta Endocrinol. (Kbh),* 82:449–459.
70. Thorner, M. O., Chait, A., Aitken, M., Benker, G., Bloom, S. R., Mortimer, C. H., Sanders, P., Stuart Mason, A., and Besser, G. M. (1975): Bromocriptine treatment of acromegaly. *Br. Med. J.,* 1:299–303.
71. Thorner, M. O., Ryan, S. M., Wass, J. A. H., Jones, A., Bouloux, P., Williams, S., and Besser, G. M. (1978): Effect of the dopamine agonist, lergotrile mesylate, and circulating anterior pituitary hormones in man. *J. Clin. Endocrinol. Metab.,* 47:372–378.
72. U, H. S., Wilson, C. B., and Tyrell, J. B. (1977): Transsphenoidal microhypophysectomy in acromegaly. *J. Neurosurg.,* 47:840–852.

73. Verde, G., Oppizzi, G., Colussi, G., Cremascoli, G., Botalla, L., Muller, E. E., Silvestrini, F., Chiodini, P. G., and Liuzzi, A. (1976): Effect of dopamine infusion on plasma levels of growth hormone in normal subjects and in acromegalic patients. *Clin. Endocrinol. (Oxf.),* 5:419–423.
74. Wass, J. A. H., Moult, P. J. A., Thorner, M. O., Dacie, J. E., Charlesworth, M., Jones, A. E., and Besser, G. M. (1979): Reduction of pituitary tumor size in patients with prolactinomas and acromegaly treated with bromocriptine with or without radiotherapy. *Lancet,* 2:66–69.
75. Wass, J. A. H., Thorner, M. O., Morris, D. V., Rees, L. H., Stuart Mason, A., Jones, A., and Besser, G. M. (1977): Long-term treatment of acromegaly with bromocriptine. *Br. Med. J.,* 1:875–878.
76. Werner, S., Hall, K., and Sjöberg, H. E. (1978): Bromocriptine therapy in patients with acromegaly: Effects on growth hormone, somatomedin A, and prolactin. *Acta Endocrinol.* 88(Suppl. 216):199–206.
77. Williams, R. A., Jacobs, H. S., Kurtz, A. B., Millar, J. S. B., Oakley, N. W., Spathis, G. S., Sullway, M. J., and Nabarro, J. D. N. (1975): The treatment of acromegaly with special reference to trans-sphenoidal hypophysectomy. *Q. J. Med.,* 44:79–98.
78. Wilson, C. B., and Dempsey, L. C. (1978): Transsphenoidal microsurgical removal of 250 pituitary adenomas. *J. Neurosurg.,* 48:13–22.
79. Winkelman, W., Schran, H., Hadam, W. R., Hessen, D., and Mies, R. (1975): Effects of apomorphine and cyproheptadine on GH and PRL in normals and in acromegaly. *International Symposium on Growth Hormone and Related Peptides,* Milan, Abstract 99.
80. Woolf, P. D., and Lee, L. (1977): Effect of the serotonin precursor, tryptophan, on pituitary hormone secretion. *J. Clin. Endocrinol. Metab.,* 45:123–133.
81. Wright, A. D., Hill, D. M., Lowy, C., and Russel Fraser, T. (1970): Mortality in acromegaly. *Q. J. Med.,* 39:1–16.

5

Bromocriptine Therapy for Parkinsonism

I. INTRODUCTION

Parkinsonism is one of the most common neurological disorders. The salient clinical features are tremor, rigidity, and reduced, slow, clumsy movement (hypokinesia; bradykinesia). The prevalence of parkinsonism in Europe and North America is about 1 in 1,000, but in subjects over 60 years of age this figure rises to 1 in 100. Although certain drugs (particularly phenothiazines), toxic agents, and infections can induce a parkinsonian syndrome, in the vast majority of cases no causal agent can be identified; this form of the disorder is termed idiopathic parkinsonism, paralysis agitans, or Parkinson's disease.

II. ETIOLOGY OF PARKINSONISM

There are not many clues to the etiology of Parkinson's disease. Its relationship to the process of aging of the nervous system has been an enigma that has stimulated a number of studies. With advancing age a range of morphological, biochemical, physiological, and psychological changes occur, and many of these trends are seen in an exaggerated form in Parkinson's disease. Examples are loss of dopaminergic neurons, dopamine, enzymes and cofactors involved in producing dopamine, long loop reflexes, external ocular movements, manual dexterity, and intellectual performance. This list is certainly incomplete, but its extension will still leave unanswered the tantalizing question of how Parkinson's disease comes to represent such a caricature of the profile of neurological deterioration in late life.

Patients with Parkinson's disease occasionally have a family history of the disorder, and the pattern of involvement in these cases indicates an autosomal dominant inheritance. Parkinsonism is less common in black subjects, but no adequate explanation has been put forward to explain this epidemiological finding. One of the few environmental factors to have been established as bearing on parkinsonism is an inverse relationship with smoking.

While the cause of parkinsonism remains obscure, it is known that the syndrome is associated with decreased dopaminergic transmission in the basal ganglia. There appears to be a somewhat selective degeneration of the dopaminergic nigrostriatal tract, leading to depletion of dopamine but leaving the striatal dopamine receptors intact. Indeed, there seems to be an increase of dopamine receptors, which has been attributed to induction of denervation supersensitivity (14). Postmortem examination of parkinsonian brains indicates that the loss of dopamine has already reached substantial proportions by the time the clinical features appear, and it may be inferred that significantly enhanced striatal sensitivity to dopamine has already developed. These findings have important therapeutic implications:

(a) The loss of dopaminergic nigral cells leads to a reduction in the concentration of enzymes responsible for synthesizing dopamine—tyrosine hydroxylase and L-aromatic aminoacid decarboxylase. Administration of precursors of dopamine can therefore be predicted to generate only incomplete restoration of dopamine levels in the brain.

(b) Conversely, the induction of dopaminergic receptor supersensitivity can be expected to result in an augmented response to dopaminergic drugs. In particular, tissue concentrations of dopaminergic agents that are insufficient to affect transmission at normal dopaminergic synapses are likely to facilitate transmission at sites involved by the neuropathology and denervation supersensitivity of parkinsonism. This situation is conducive to eliciting a high therapeutic index—dopaminergic drugs should act preferentially at sites where they are needed, without concomitantly producing side effects by disturbing transmission elsewhere.

III. THE NEED FOR NEW THERAPY

Following the discovery that dopamine is depleted from the brains of parkinsonian patients, it was suggested that deficient dopaminergic transmission might contribute to the clinical features of the disorder. Since dopamine does not readily cross the blood-brain barrier, its precursor, levodopa, was investigated as a possible therapeutic agent. Initially, small doses of 100 to 200 mg were administered, and equivocal observations were reported. However, in 1967 Cotzias and colleagues (2) found that the emesis normally encountered with higher doses of levodopa could be overcome by increasing the intake of the drug very slowly. On 6 to 8 g of levodopa daily, substantial and sometimes dramatic improvement of parkinsonism was achieved (2). The majority of patients responded, and benefit was seen in all of the neurological deficits associated with the syndrome. Like most powerful drugs, however, levodopa induced prominent adverse reactions. Emesis remained one of the common early side effects of levodopa therapy.

This anorexia, nausea, and vomiting appeared to derive from the conversion of levodopa to catecholamines outside the blood-brain barrier, probably through stimulation of the chemoreceptor trigger zone in the medulla oblongata. In 1971, this problem was alleviated but not eliminated by concomitant administration of carbidopa or benserazide. These agents blocked the enzyme converting levodopa to dopamine (L-aromatic aminoacid decarboxylase), but they were unable to cross the blood-brain barrier, so levodopa could still be transformed to dopamine where it was needed, in the striatum (25).

Following the introduction of extracerebral decarboxylase inhibitors, a period of satisfactory therapy emerged for most parkinsonian patients. This lasted 3 to 6 years, after which time a progressively increasing proportion of patients began to encounter serious difficulties (5). These included declining efficacy, increasing choreoathetoid movements (dyskinesia), dementia, and severe fluctuations in response from phases resembling florid levodopa overdosage to periods of profound underdosage. In some patients these oscillations in performance were related to the timing of doses ("wearing off" reactions and "end of dose" akinesia). In other patients the dramatic and often devastating fluctuations were unrelated to the time of levodopa intake ("on-off" reactions).

The basis of these various problems remains obscure, but it became clear that new concepts of treatment were desirable. A number of methods are now available for predicting the possible antiparkinsonism efficacy of newly synthesized compounds.

A. Strategies for Developing Antiparkinsonism Therapy

The oldest effective treatment for parkinsonism was blockade of muscarinic cholinergic receptors. A century ago, the efficacy of belladonna alkaloids was discovered by chance; over 50 years were to elapse before it was recognized that these drugs achieved their pharmacological effect by antagonizing the muscarinic effects of acetylcholine. Later, after the recognition of the crucial importance of decreased dopaminergic transmission in parkinsonism, the beneficial action of anticholinergic drugs was attributed to restoration of neurotransmitter balance in a setting where dopamine and acetylcholine elicited antagonistic effects in the basal ganglia.

The era of rational development of pharmacotherapy for parkinsonism has been characterized by the development of test systems for evaluating the dopaminergic properties of newly synthesized compounds. Dopaminergic screening has been reviewed in some detail in Chapter 1, so it will merely be summarized here.

In vitro tests include studies on synaptosomal preparations or brain slices to detect the release of dopamine or the blockade of its reuptake. In homogenates of caudate tissue, the formation of cyclic adenosine monophosphate (cAMP) has been employed as a method of assessing dopaminergic properties. However, it has now been recognized that this response is elicited by one category of receptors (termed D-1), whereas another receptor type (termed D-2) can be activated without any change in cAMP levels. The best *in vitro* test for activation of D-2 receptors is probably inhibition of the release of prolactin from preparations of anterior pituitary cells *(see Chapter 1).*

In vivo tests are more numerous. Reduction of prolactin levels in the plasma is a sensitive way to detect dopaminergic activity. Other tests include measurement of: increased locomotor activity; stereotypic behavior; induction of rotation after placing unilateral lesions in the substantia nigra; decreased body temperature in a cold environment; reversal of the reserpine syndrome; inhibition of brain synthesis of dopamine; and reduction in the electrical activity of dopaminergic neurons. Rats are employed in all of these methods. In primates, experimental lesions of the brain stem produce tremor, which is alleviated by dopaminergic agents.

With all of these techniques available, it is not surprising that numerous dopamine receptor agonists have been identified. However, there are serious limitations in the application of these test systems to the development of new antiparkinsonism agents. For example, it is not known which tests correlate best with therapeutic efficacy and which predict unwanted dopaminergic effects, such as dyskinesia or psychosis. These questions will be answered only when more laboratory and clinical evidence is available on a wide range of compounds, so that profiles of pharmacological activity can be matched with a diversity of responses in patients.

B. Dopamine Receptor Agonists

One approach to the current problems encountered with levodopa therapy is the development of drugs that mimic dopamine at the receptor–dopamine agonists (DA). Theoretically, an ideal artificial agonist of dopamine might be developed with the following advantages over levodopa:

1. By acting directly on dopaminergic receptors, an artificial agonist would bypass the need for L-aromatic aminoacid decarboxylase (as already mentioned, this enzyme, required for the conversion of levodopa to dopamine, is depleted in the brains of parkinsonian patients).
2. Administration of levodopa leads to modification of function in noradrenergic and serotonergic synapses; an artificial agonist should be specific for dopamine receptors. Furthermore, as already mentioned, it is likely that there exist multiple categories of dopamine receptors and that therapeutic effects may stem from activation at only one type *(see below)*. Adverse reactions may result from stimulation of other types of dopamine receptors. Hence, the possibility of introducing increased specificity, with an appropriate agonist, offers a chance of decreasing some of the centrally induced adverse reactions to levodopa.
3. The half-life of levodopa is short in the plasma (about 1½ hr). A dopamine agonist with a longer half-life might be predicted to smooth out the response in those patients with "wearing off" reactions or "end of dose" akinesia.

For these reasons, the quest for a suitable dopamine agonist has been pressed in an attempt to improve treatment for parkinsonism. The first such drug to be tried was apomorphine, which had therapeutic properties but proved to be nephrotoxic. A congener, *N*-propylnoraporphine, was also efficacious and caused less renal damage, but it was still too toxic to justify extensive study. Another dopamine agonist, piribedil, alleviated parkinsonism but produced psychiatric reactions in an unacceptably high proportion of patients.

The newest group of dopamine agonists are ergot derivatives. Of these, lergotrile has been shown to be a potent antiparkinsonism agent (16), but impairment of hepatic function occurred in some 50% of patients receiving this drug (20), so its use has been abandoned. The most satisfactory dopamine agonist to emerge for the treatment of parkinsonism is bromocriptine. Even this drug, however, has significant limitations *(see below).*

C. Dopamine Receptors and Parkinsonism

Reference has already been made to a recent subdivision of dopamine receptors into D-1 and D-2 categories (12). Current findings suggest that defective dopaminergic transmission in parkinsonism predominately involves D-2 receptors. There may even be a reciprocal relationship between D-1 and D-2 receptor systems.

The argument implicating the D-2 receptors in parkinsonism derives from the following observations:

1. Dopaminergic ergot derivatives, including bromocriptine, are potent agonists for D-2 receptors (Figs. 1 and 2), whereas in certain test systems they antagonize D-1 receptors (Fig. 2). Lergotrile has been used as an example in Figs. 1 and 2, as it is water soluble, which facilitated the performance of these experiments. Dopaminergic ergots are active antiparkinsonian agents (Fig. 3).
2. No selective D-1 agonists are available, but it may be inferred that drugs that antagonize phosphodiesterase, such as caffeine, lead to the accumulation of cAMP and hence facilitate transmission at D-1 receptors. Caffeine exacerbates parkinsonism (Fig. 4).

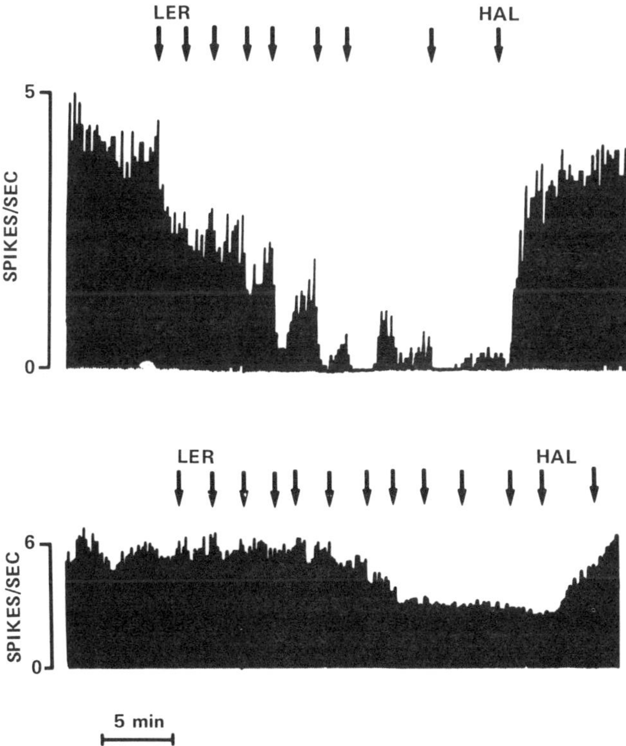

FIG. 1. Effect of i.v. administration of lergotrile (LER) and haloperidol (HAL) on firing rates of dopamine neurons in the pars compacta of the substantia nigra. **Top:** Lergotrile, administered in increasing doses (6.2, 6.2, 12.5, 25, 50, 100, 200, and 400 μg/kg), at times indicated by the arrows, progressively inhibited the firing rate of this cell until the cell ceased firing for approximately 2 min after cumulative doses of 400 and 800 μg/kg. Haloperidol (0.1 mg/kg) reversed the effects of lergotrile. **Bottom:** Lergotrile, administered in increasing doses (1.5, 1.5, 3.1, 6.2, 12.5, 25, 50, 100, 200, 400, and 800 μg/kg), inhibited the firing rate of this cell by 50%. Haloperidol (0.1, 0.2 mg/kg) reversed the effect of lergotrile. (Reproduced with permission from Walters et al., ref. 23).

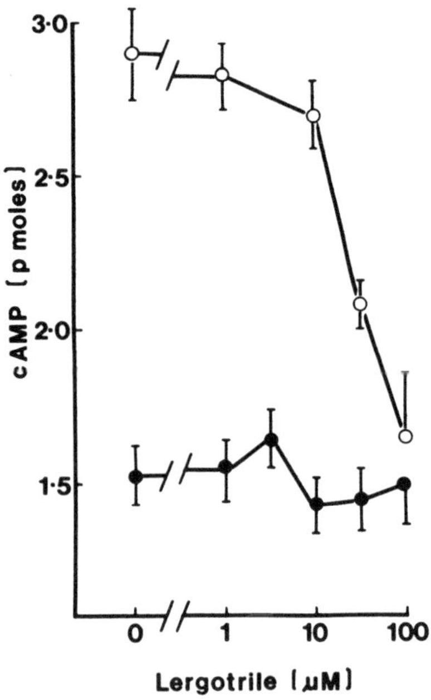

FIG. 2. Effects of lergotrile on the dopamine-stimulated adenylate cyclase activity in homogenates of rat caudate nucleus. Cyclase activity is shown in the absence (●—●) or in the presence (○—○) of 100 μM dopamine. Data represent mean ± SEM for 6 (no lergotrile) or 3 (added lergotrile) determinations of enzyme activity in replicate aliquots of a single striatal homogenate. (Reproduced with permission from Kebabian et al., ref. 13).

3. Certain dopaminergic blocking drugs, such as molindone and metoclopramide, are selective antagonists at the D-2 receptor (12). These agents can induce parkinsonism.

These observations are summarized in Table 1.

In the context of attributing clinical phenomena to predominant involvement of D-1 or D-2 receptors, it is of interest to mention that dopaminergic ergots (bromocriptine and lergotrile) that stimulate D-2 receptors selectively produce adverse reactions, which include schizophrenic psychosis. Correspondingly, selective an-

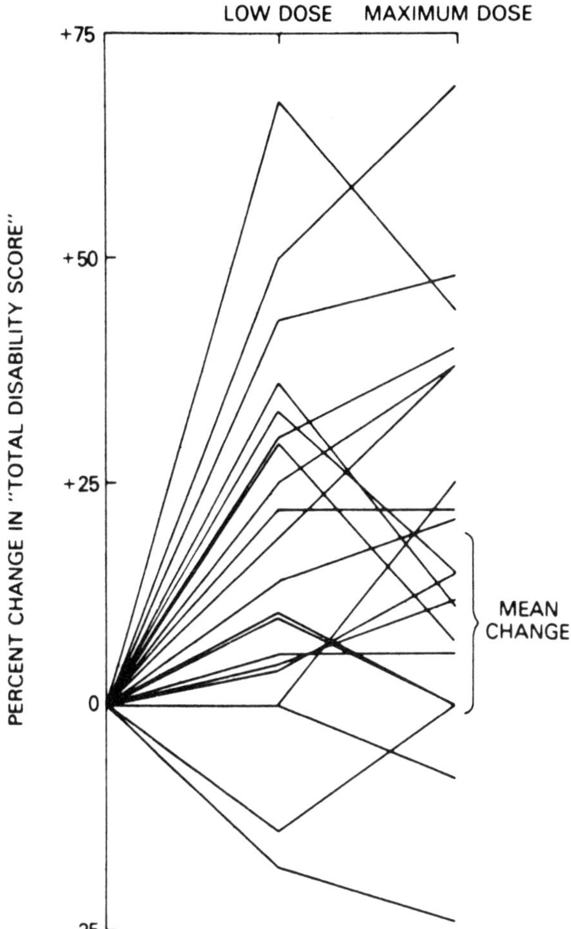

FIG. 3. "Total disability score" in 20 patients treated with bromocriptine. Lines represent the change in each patient during the phases of treatment with bromocriptine. Positive values indicate an improvement and negative values indicate a deterioration. (Reproduced with permission from Kartzinel et al., ref. 10.)

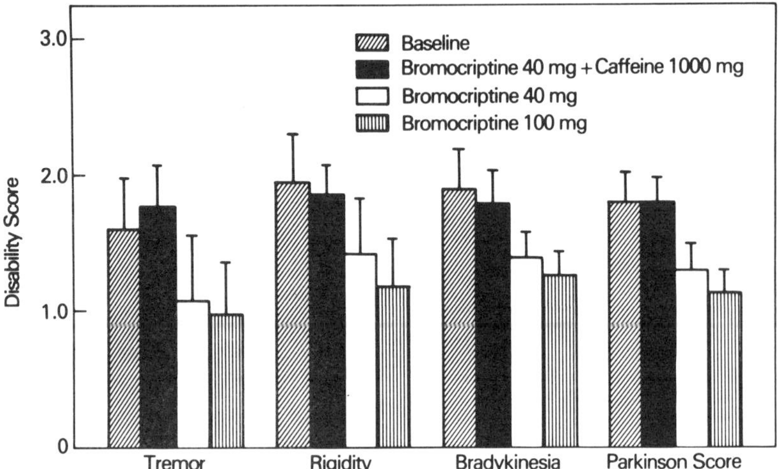

FIG. 4. Clinical response to caffeine (1,000 mg daily) and bromocriptine (40 and 100 mg daily) in 6 patients with idiopathic parkinsonism. The "baseline" values represent scores obtained when patients were receiving optimal conventional therapy (including levodopa). The "Parkinson score" was computed by taking the average of the disability scores for tremor, rigidity, and bradykinesia. The standard error of the mean is represented by vertical lines. (Reproduced with permission from Kartzinel et al., ref. 11.)

tagonists of D-2 receptors (such as molindone) are employed as therapeutic agents in the management of schizophrenia. These findings implicate excessive D-2 activation as one possible factor contributing to schizophrenia.

TABLE 1. *Relationship between parkinsonism and drugs influencing dopamine receptors*

	D_1	D_2	Parkinsonism
DA ergots	−	+	Improved
Caffeine	+	0	Exacerbated
Molindone	0	−	Exacerbated

IV. BROMOCRIPTINE THERAPY

A. In Parkinsonism

Bromocriptine emerged from laboratory evaluation as a substance of sufficient dopaminergic specificity and potency to merit investigation as a potential therapeutic tool in parkinsonism. Biochemical observations indicate that bromocriptine acts as a dopamine agonist in the central nervous system in man; its administration leads to a reduction in the concentration of homovanillic acid (Fig. 5). Such a finding is generally accepted as evidence for activation of presynaptic dopamine receptors, leading to decreased release of transmitter.

Numerous clinical studies have been undertaken to assess bromocriptine in Parkinson's disease (1,3,4,6–8,10,15,17,18). Initial results were conflicting, a predictable outcome since the doses of bromocriptine given in different investigations ranged from 15 to 150 mg daily.

When bromocriptine was first employed in parkinsonism, evidence from its use in human endocrinological diseases indicated that 15 mg daily was more than adequate to induce complete suppression of prolactin release. It was therefore anticipated that 15 mg daily would be sufficient to elicit an antiparkinsonian effect, if the drug possessed such a property. However, a daily intake of 15 mg bromocriptine yielded equivocal findings. Because of the analogy with the slight therapeutic response seen a decade earlier with low doses of levodopa, an effort was made to increase the dose of bromocriptine. Substantial efficacy was detected at higher doses, but adverse reactions became much more frequent when the daily intake reached 100 to 150 mg. It is not clear why higher doses of bromocriptine are required to treat parkinsonism, compared with hyperprolactinemia; one relevant factor may be that the blood-brain barrier impedes access of drugs to the striatum, whereas there is no such hindrance in the case of the pituitary.

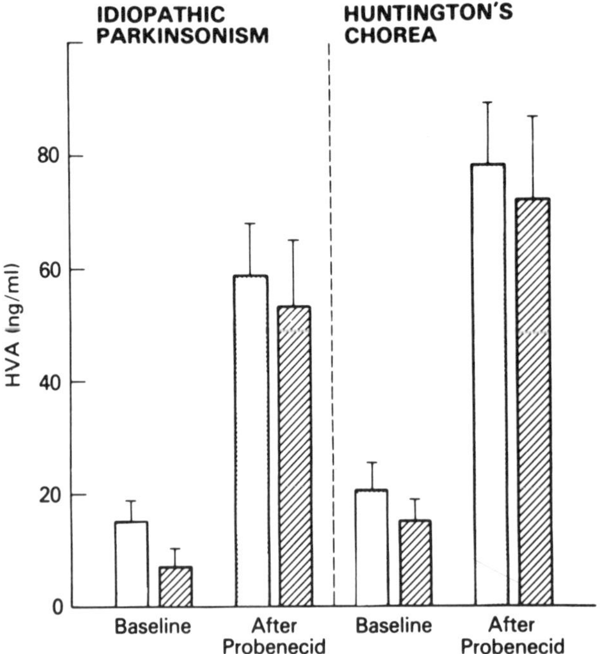

FIG. 5. Effects of chronic bromocriptine therapy (up to 100 mg daily) on CSF monoamine metabolites in 6 patients with parkinsonism and 6 with Huntington's chorea. Results both with and without prior infusion of probenecid (40 mg/kg over 1 hr). (Data from Kartzinel et al., ref. 9.)

In addition to variation in dosage contributing to the controversial reports on bromocriptine, other relevant factors included the variation in types of patient and the management of concomitant treatment with other drugs. Thus, some studies comprised mildly disabled patients, whereas others included subjects with severe disease; certain trials involved patients with "on-off" reactions, and others selected patients who showed no response to levodopa. In some studies, patients were not receiving levodopa, in others the levodopa dose was unaltered, and in still others, the dose of levodopa was reduced substantially while the dose of bromocriptine was increased. A further important variable compounding the confusion was the duration of treatment with bromocriptine, which ranged from 2 weeks to 2 years. From such a wide variety of studies it is scarcely surprising that reports ranged from unbridled enthusiasm to profound pessimism. Now that a reasonably extensive collective clinical experience has accrued, it is possible to discuss some meaningful patterns in the results, which allow certain generalizations to be made without bias or excessive oversimplification.

1. Bromocriptine is an effective antiparkinsonian agent that is useful in the management of some, but not all, parkinsonian patients.
2. In parkinsonism, the optimal dose range of bromocriptine is 40 to 80 mg daily.
3. To minimize adverse reactions, the dose of bromocriptine should be built up gradually over a period of 6 to 8 weeks. It is desirable to give an initial test dose of 1 mg, because occasional patients are extremely sensitive to the hypotensive action of bromocriptine.
4. Another important factor in reducing unwanted effects is reduction of the dose of levodopa in patients who are already taking this drug. It is usually desirable to cut the intake of levodopa by some 50%. This decrease should be effected gradually, while the dose of bromocriptine is being increased.
5. All the clinical features of parkinsonism may be alleviated by bromocriptine, but its main advantage is the lower incidence and decreased severity of dyskinesia (when compared with levodopa). Bromocriptine also has a more protracted action than levodopa, possibly because of its longer plasma half-life *(see Chapter 2).*
6. The major problem with bromocriptine is induction of psychiatric reactions, which include confusion, hallucinations, and delusions. These effects are similar to those encountered with levodopa, but when such symptoms arise in patients taking bromocriptine, they are generally more severe and may last longer. Adverse reactions to bromocriptine are discussed in more detail

in Chapter 6, but in addition to psychiatric problems, it is appropriate here to mention hypotension, cardiac arrhythmia, and erythromelalgia.

7. Many patients fail to achieve sustained benefit from bromocriptine, or experience intolerable adverse reactions, so that only about 50% continue to take the drug over prolonged periods.

8. The high doses of bromocriptine that are employed for long-term treatment of parkinsonism present a significant economic burden; bromocriptine is considerably more expensive than any other antiparkinsonian drug.

Bromocriptine can be given in combination with any of the various drugs employed to treat parkinsonism, such as levodopa, carbidopa, benserazide, amantadine, anticholinergic agents, and antihistaminic drugs. One recent development of considerable interest is the combination of bromocriptine with a dopamine antagonist that does not cross the blood-brain barrier. Initial reports with a peripheral dopamine blocker, domperidone, suggest that concomitant administration of bromocriptine with this drug leads to a substantial improvement in the therapeutic index over that attainable with bromocriptine alone, or with bromocriptine plus levodopa. It is desirable to have confirmation and extension of these findings.

The process of starting bromocriptine therapy in patients already receiving levodopa is an arduous trial of the patient's tenacity and the physician's skill. Numerous outpatient consultations are required, at which detailed instructions must be given on the dual problem of slowly raising the intake of bromocriptine and simultaneously reducing the levodopa. Charts of the regimen recommended for each day over a 2-week period are helpful, at the end of which time it is normally necessary to review the patient's progress and reevaluate the dose schedule. The problem is one of continually titrating dosage against adverse reactions on one hand, and inadequate control of parkinsonism on the other. After a 1 mg test dose, it is reasonable to start patients on 2.5 mg t.i.d., initially increasing by 2.5 mg every 2 to 3 days.

On reaching 20 mg daily, 5 mg increments can be employed. When a maintenance regimen is reached, it is convenient to divide the daily intake into four or five approximately equal doses.

Treatment of patients who are not receiving levodopa is easier, since only one drug dose has to be adjusted. It is of considerable interest that the use of bromocriptine in patients who have never received levodopa leads to a therapeutic response in which dyskinesia is very seldom encountered—although this adverse reaction is the commonest dose-limiting problem in patients who are taking levodopa.

Bromocriptine is contraindicated in patients with a history of psychiatric symptoms (confusion, hallucinations, or delusions), a recent myocardial infarction (or other cardiac lesion predisposing to an arrhythmia), or peripheral vascular disease. Reasons for stopping bromocriptine therapy in Parkinson's disease include the appearance of psychotic symptoms, development of an erythromelalgia-like syndrome, induction of a cardiac arrhythmia, or the emergence of ergotism.

From this review, the current status of bromocriptine in the treatment of parkinsonism can be summarized as follows:

1. Bromocriptine is helpful in certain patients. It is usually desirable to give it in combination with submaximal doses of levodopa. The role of bromocriptine has appropriately been referred to by Parkes as "a refinement, rather than replacement of levodopa therapy."

2. Bromocriptine represents a new approach to treating parkinsonism. Its success, together with its limitations, affords support for the quest for other dopaminergic agonists that will provide increased efficacy with less toxicity.

B. In Other Extrapyramidal Disorders

There have been a number of reports that low doses of dopamine agonists, such as apomorphine and bromocriptine, can alleviate other extrapyramidal disorders, notably Huntington's chorea and tardive dyskinesia (19,21,22). Such findings are of considerable theoretical interest, since they support the suggestion, deriving from laboratory studies, that low concentrations of bromocriptine stimulate presynaptic receptors selectively and thus lead to a decreased release of dopamine. However, from a practical viewpoint these findings are unlikely to have any major impact upon the management of Huntington's disease or tardive dyskinesia, because the therapeutic dose range is so narrow. In some patients the dose is likely to be too small to produce any effect, whereas in others there will be a risk of exacerbation of involuntary movements and augmentation of psychotic behavior.

Finally, there exist certain neurological diseases in which the symptom complex of parkinsonism comprises a portion of the total clinical picture. Such disorders include the Shy-Drager and Steele-Richardson-Olszewski syndromes. In these "paraparkinsonian" conditions, the results of bromocriptine therapy have proved disappointing, although occasionally some temporary, limited improvement has been achieved (24). In such cases, the optimal dose regimen of bromocriptine has been the same as that employed in Parkinson's disease, but in patients with Shy-Drager syndrome it has been necessary to give smaller and less frequent dosage increments when starting treatment. Therapeutic results in Shy-Drager and Steele-Richardson-Olszewski syndromes tend to occur in younger patients with mild disease, possibly because the dopaminergic receptors have not yet become seriously involved in the underlying neuropathology.

In summary, the use of bromocriptine in extrapyramidal disorders other than Parkinson's disease has yielded results that have been of interest, but of no practical importance for routine management.

REFERENCES

1. Calne, D. B., Williams, A. C., Neophytides, A., Plotkin, C., Nutt, J. G., and Teychenne, P. F. (1978): Long-term treatment of parkinsonism with bromocriptine. *Lancet,* 1:735–738.

2. Cotzias, C. G., Van Woert, M. H., and Schiffer, L. M. (1967): Aromatic amino acids and modification of parkinsonism. *N. Engl. J. Med.*, 276:374–379.
3. Debono, A. G., Marsden, C. D., Asselman, P., and Parkes, J. D. (1976): Bromocriptine and dopamine receptor stimulation. *Br. J. Clin. Pharmacol.*, 3:977–982.
4. Duvoisin, R. C., Mendoza, M. R., Yahr, M. D., and Sweet, R. D. (1979): Bromocriptine as an adjuvant to levodopa. In: *Dopaminergic Ergot Derivatives and Motor Function,* edited by K. Fuxe and D. B. Calne, pp. 329–336. Pergamon Press, Oxford.
5. Fahn, S., and Calne, D. B. (1978): Considerations in the management of parkinsonism. *Neurology,* 28:5–7.
6. Fahn, S., Cote, L. J., Snider, S. R., Barrett, R. E., and Isgreen, W. P. (1979): Role of bromocriptine in the treatment of parkinsonism. In: *Dopaminergic Ergot Derivatives and Motor Function,* edited by K. Fuxe and D. B. Calne, pp. 303–312. Pergamon Press, Oxford.
7. Godwin-Austen, R. B. (1979): Bromocriptine compared with levodopa in parkinsonism. In: *Dopaminergic Ergot Derivatives and Motor Function,* edited by K. Fuxe and D. B. Calne, pp. 297–302. Pergamon Press, Oxford.
8. Grøn, U. (1979): Clinical observations with bromocriptine in parkinsonism. In: *Dopaminergic Ergot Derivatives and Motor Function,* edited by K. Fuxe and D. B. Calne, pp. 343–348. Pergamon Press, Oxford.
9. Kartzinel, R., Perlow, M. D., Carter, A. C., Chase, T. N., Calne, D. B., and Shoulson, I. (1976): Metabolic studies with bromocriptine in patients with idiopathic parkinsonism and Huntington's chorea. *Trans. Am. Neurol. Assoc.,* 101:53–56.
10. Kartzinel, R., Perlow, M., Teychenne, P., Gielen, A. C., Gillespie, M. M., Sadowsky, D. A., and Calne, D. B. (1976): Bromocriptine and levodopa (with or without carbidopa) in parkinsonism. *Lancet,* 2:272–275.
11. Kartzinel, R., Shoulson, I., and Calne, D. B. (1976): Studies with bromocriptine. III. Concomitant administration of caffeine to patients with idiopathic parkinsonism. *Neurology,* 26:741–743.
12. Kebabian, J. W., and Calne, D. B. (1979): Multiple receptors for dopamine. *Nature,* 277:93–96.
13. Kebabian, J. W., Calne, D. B., and Kebabian, P. R. (1977): Lergotrile mesylate: An *in vivo* dopamine agonist which blocks dopamine receptors *in vitro. Commun. Psychopharmacol.,* 1:311–318.
14. Lee, T., Seeman, P., Raiput, A., Farley, I. J., and Hornykiewicz, O. (1978): Receptor basis for dopaminergic supersensitivity in Parkinson's disease. *Nature,* 273:59–61.
15. Lieberman, A. N., Kupersmith, M., Gopinathan, G., Estey, E., and Goldstein, M. (1979): Modification of the "On-Off" effect with bromocriptine and lergotrile. In: *Dopaminergic Ergot Derivatives and Motor Function,* edited by K. Fuxe and D. B. Calne, pp. 285–296. Pergamon Press, Oxford.
16. Lieberman, A., Miyamoto, T., Battista, A. F., and Goldstein, M. (1975): Studies on the antiparkinsonian efficacy of lergotrile. *Neurology,* 25:459–462.

17. Rinne, U. K., Marttila, R., and Sonninen, V. (1979): Relationship between dopamine turnover and the therapeutic response to bromocriptine. In: *Dopaminergic Ergot Derivatives and Motor Function,* edited by K. Fuxe and D. B. Calne, pp. 319–328. Pergamon Press, Oxford.
18. Stern, G., Lees, A., and Shaw, K. (1979): Ergot derivatives without levodopa in parkinsonism. In: *Dopaminergic Ergot Derivatives and Motor Function,* edited by K. Fuxe and D. B. Calne, pp. 337–342. Pergamon Press, Oxford.
19. Tamminga, C. A., Schaffer, M. H., and Chase, T. N. (1979): Ergot derivatives in the treatment of psychotic and hyperkinetic disorders. In: *Dopaminergic Ergot Derivatives and Motor Function,* edited by K. Fuxe and D. B. Calne, pp. 349–360. Pergamon Press, Oxford.
20. Teychenne, P. F., Jones, E. A., Ishak, Kamal, and Calne, D. B. (1979): Hepatocellular injury with distinctive mitochondrial changes induced by lergotrile mesylate: A dopaminergic ergot derivative. *Gastroenterology,* 76:575–583.
21. Tolosa, E. S., and Sparber, S. B. (1974): Bromocriptine in Huntington's chorea. *Arch. Neurol.,* 33:517–518.
22. Trabucchi, M., Albizzati, M. G., Spano, P. F., Tonon, G., and Frattola, L. (1979): Ergot derivatives in dyskinetic and dystonic disorders. In: *Dopaminergic Ergot Derivatives and Motor Function,* edited by K. Fuxe and D. B. Calne, pp. 361–369. Pergamon Press, Oxford.
23. Walters, J. R., Lakoski, J. M., Baring, M. D., and Eng, N. (1979): Dopamine neurons: Effect of lergotrile on unit activity and transmitter synthesis. *Eur. J. Pharmacol.,* 60:199–210.
24. Williams, A. C., Nutt, J., Lake, C. R., Pfeiffer, R., Teychenne, P. E., Ebert, M., and Calne, D. B. (1979): Actions of bromocriptine in the Shy-Drager and Steele-Richardson-Olszewski syndromes. In: *Dopaminergic Ergot Derivatives and Motor Function,* edited by K. Fuxe and D. B. Calne, pp. 271–284. Pergamon Press, Oxford.
25. Yahr, M. D., editor (1973): *Treatment of Parkinsonism—The Role of Dopa Decarboxylase Inhibitors. Advances in Neurology, Vol. 2.* Raven Press, New York.

6

Adverse Reactions to Bromocriptine

There is little doubt that bromocriptine is an extremely useful addition to therapeutics. Its place in the management of both neuroendocrine and neurological disease remains to be clearly defined, as discussed in Chapters 3, 4, 5, and 7. However, adverse effects do occur and although none appears to cause permanent damage, they should be understood by both the physician and the patient in order that they may be minimized or, preferably,

TABLE 1. *Adverse effects of bromocriptine*

Adverse effects associated with the initiation of therapy
nausea
vomiting
postural hypotension
Adverse effects of chronic therapy
In all groups of subjects
headaches and nasal stuffiness
gastrointestinal: dyspepsia, constipation, GI bleeding
cold–sensitive digital vasospasm
alcohol intolerance
increased arousal
In parkinsonism only
dyskinesia
psychiatric disorders
erythromelalgia
Toxicologic considerations

prevented entirely. It is difficult to be certain of the true incidence of adverse reactions, as reporting depends to a large extent on the care and detail of the studies being performed. However, clinicians agree that patients with certain diseases are more sensitive to side effects than are others. Furthermore, some adverse reactions are seen only with very high doses and others are seen only in patients with certain conditions—for example, psychiatric side effects in parkinsonian patients.

Two major groups of side effects have been described (Table 1). The first are seen with the initiation of therapy, and the second during long-term administration. Both groups of adverse reactions are well described with the use of levodopa and presumably reflect widespread stimulation of central and peripheral dopamine receptors. In contrast, cold-sensitive digital vasospasm, erythromelalgia, alcohol intolerance, and gastrointestinal bleeding seem to be specific to bromocriptine. At higher doses, bromocriptine may have pharmacologic actions apart from stimulation of dopamine receptors.

I. ADVERSE REACTIONS WITH INITIATION OF THERAPY

A. Nausea, Vomiting, and Postural Hypotension

The incidence of nausea, vomiting, and postural hypotension during initiation of therapy varies with the condition for which the patient is being treated. Young, normal subjects taking bromocriptine experimentally for the purposes of clinical research appear to be particularly susceptible. Patients with hyperprolactinemia are also fairly sensitive, whereas those with acromegaly only rarely have severe initial side effects. Similarly, these side effects have only rarely been reported in women given bromocriptine to suppress postpartum lactation. However, in all groups of patients these adverse reactions may be minimized or prevented by giving a small dose with food on their retiring at night. If the patient remains recumbent, the nausea and vomiting can be obviated, and in this position the hypotension is not seen. Food appears to slow absorption of the drug, and thus the stimulation to dopamine receptors may be more gradual and less profound (7). The dose is then gradually increased over 24 to 72 hr by adding an extra dose—for example, 1.25 mg once daily—then by increasing the dose to two times, then three times, and finally, if indicated, to four times daily. The dose is then raised to 2.5 mg at each time, building up over a space of 1 to 3 weeks to the required maintenance dose. The speed with which the dose can be escalated varies from patient to patient, and therefore it is essential that both the physician and patient understand that the side effects are transient and dose-related. If adverse reactions occur, the dose can be maintained or reduced as required, and if necessary the drug can be stopped. On recommencing therapy in a patient who has suffered from side effects, the dose should be escalated more slowly and the initial dose should be lower. Sometimes the adverse reactions cannot be avoided, but continuation of therapy leads to tolerance to these unwanted effects, although therapeutic efficacy is not compromised.

Patients who are treated for disorders of prolactin secretion rarely require more than 7.5 mg/day (low dose), whereas those with acromegaly and parkinsonism require from 10 to 80 mg/day. With the "low-dose" regimen, only the minor adverse effects of starting treatment occur.

II. ADVERSE REACTIONS WITH CHRONIC THERAPY

A. In All Groups of Patients

Adverse reactions do not, in general, present serious problems or prevent continuation of therapy in patients on low doses for hyperprolactinemia. In contrast, high-dose bromocriptine treatment of acromegaly and parkinsonism is associated with an appreciable incidence of major side effects. Only rarely do they prevent continuation of therapy in acromegalic patients; in parkinsonism, where the adverse reactions are more profound, discontinuation of therapy may be necessary. Dyskinesia, psychiatric disorders, erythromelalgia, transient elevation of hepatic enzymes, and cardiac dysrhythmias have been seen only in parkinsonian patients. Parkinsonian patients represent an older and sicker population, with widespread disease and often with unassociated pathology, e.g., ischemic heart disease. Thus, the side effects seen in these patients are a result of reduced compensatory reserve for the pharmacologic effects of the drug as compared to that of patients with isolated pituitary disease. It is possible that, for example, the increased arousal seen in a few acromegalic patients may be the counterpart of the psychiatric disturbance in parkinsonian patients. All untoward reactions may be reversed by withdrawing or lowering the dose of the drug.

1. Headaches and Nasal Stuffiness

Mild headaches and nasal stuffiness commonly occur at the start of bromocriptine therapy. They are seldom severe and are often transitory.

2. Gastrointestinal Side Effects

Apart from the nausea and vomiting mentioned above, which may be seen with the initiation of therapy, gastrointestinal side effects are unusual.

Dyspepsia occurs occasionally during high-dose therapy. It is brought on by lying flat or by bending down. The symptoms are typical of esophageal reflux. It is possible that bromocriptine may relax the physiologic cardiac sphincter, since metoclopramide, a dopamine antagonist, increases the tone in this sphincter (10).

Constipation occurs in approximately 50% of acromegalic patients taking bromocriptine (2,9,13), and in almost all parkinsonian patients. In parkinsonism it is difficult to relate this to bromocriptine, since constipation is a symptom of parkinsonism and a complication of all antiparkinsonian therapies. In a proportion of acromegalic patients, continuation of the drug leads to resolution of this symptom; if it does not resolve, it can be simply treated with a bulk laxative.

Gastrointestinal bleeding from peptic ulceration has been described in 6 of 96 acromegalic patients receiving bromocriptine (12). The natural incidence of gastrointestinal bleeding in this group is unclear. However, in all 6 patients the bleeding was severe and the question has arisen whether or not the vascular hemostatic response to the bleeding may have been impaired by bromocriptine (12).

3. Cold-Sensitive Digital Vasospasm

Cold-sensitive digital vasospasm was initially seen only when patients were treated long-term with high-dose bromocriptine. It occurs in approximately 30% of acromegalic patients (2,6,11) and has also been reported in parkinsonian patients (3). It is not true "ergotism," since it is painless, has never led to ischemia of the phalanges, and can be reversed by lowering the dose. It may be prevented by keeping the fingers warm.

4. Alcohol Intolerance

Fewer than 10% of acromegalic patients noted that they could not tolerate their usual alcohol intake when starting on bromocriptine therapy. However, with continued therapy this effect waned (13).

5. Increased Arousal and Leg Cramps

Rarely, patients treated with high-dose bromocriptine for acromegaly noted that they required less sleep and became more active. This side effect is seldom a problem and in fact most patients are delighted with this effect, which they consider advantageous. A few patients have also complained of cramps in the calves of their legs, which appear to be related to bromocriptine therapy. However, this was not a major problem.

B. In Parkinsonism Only

1. Dyskinesia

Choreoathetoid involuntary movements (dyskinesia) of the limbs and axial musculature (including the head and neck) are characteristic manifestations of levodopa overdosage in parkinsonian patients. Indeed, these movements are by far the most common dose-limiting adverse reaction to levodopa therapy. Although the movements are most frequently of a choreic or athetoid nature, they can display the features of almost any motor disorder, including dystonia and myoclonus.

The mechanism of induction of dyskinesia is not understood. It is notable that experimental studies with levodopa in normal subjects and depressed patients have failed to record dyskinesia as an adverse reaction. It has therefore been suggested that the neuropathology of parkinsonism leads to denervation supersensitivity at striatal dopaminergic receptors, which allows levodopa to generate dyskinesia as a toxic motor reaction. In support of this view, dyskinesia tends to become more prominent as the severity of the parkinsonian syndrome advances.

In parkinsonian patients who have previously been treated with levodopa and have developed dyskinesia, the same movements can be induced by bromocriptine, irrespective of whether or not they continue to receive levodopa. However, the movements induced by bromocriptine are less severe than those generated by high doses of levodopa.

Of particular interest is a recent report that parkinsonian patients who have not previously been exposed to levodopa do not develop dyskinesia as an adverse reaction to bromocriptine (8). Although experience with such patients is limited, it will be of considerable importance to extend these observations and follow the long-term course of parkinsonian patients who have never been treated with levodopa.

From a practical viewpoint, most parkinsonian patients receiving bromocriptine will have previously encountered dyskinesia induced by levodopa. In such patients, the dose of bromocriptine must be reevaluated every 2 or 3 months so that the intake of dopaminergic drugs can be reduced if dyskinesia is prominent.

2. *Psychiatric Reactions*

Advanced, untreated Parkinson's disease can be associated with depression, dementia, hallucinations, and delusions (5). Any antiparkinsonian therapy can elicit or exacerbate these problems. Probably, as many as 20% of patients on anticholinergic drugs experience adverse psychiatric effects. The prevalence may be similar for patients receiving levodopa; there is a particular tendency for this drug to cause hallucinations and paranoid delusions. With bromocriptine there is an even higher risk of psychotic reactions.

The earliest feature of psychiatric toxicity to levodopa or bromocriptine is usually frequent and vivid dreaming. This progresses to nocturnal hallucinations, and ultimately a highly organized delusional system develops, which is associated with visual hallucinations and paranoid ideation.

Psychiatric reactions to bromocriptine are almost entirely confined to parkinsonian patients and seem to correlate with the severity of neurological disability. Withdrawal of dopaminergic therapy is always followed by improvement in the mental state, but a return to normal may take several weeks. In some patients, discontinuing levodopa or bromocriptine leads to such profound deterioration of their parkinsonism that survival may be threatened by aspiration or by such profound decrepitude that decubitus ulceration, deep vein thrombosis, or chronic urinary infection develop. In such cases, the physician is faced with the frustrating task of titrating medications to sustain an optimal but still unsatisfactory balance between parkinsonism and psychosis.

3. *Erythromelalgia*

Patients receiving bromocriptine can develop a syndrome of red, tender, edematous extremities, often associated with a sensation of localized burning or tingling discomfort. These symptoms and signs usually start in the feet, but may extend up to the knee; they occasionally occur in the hands. There is rarely additional polyarthralgia, with elevation of the sedimentation rate. Histological examination of the affected skin reveals a low-grade vasculopathy characterized by mononuclear infiltration of the walls of dermal blood vessels (4).

This erythromelalgic syndrome is confined to parkinsonian patients receiving a prolonged, high dosage of bromocriptine, in whom the prevalence is 5 to 10%. It clears exceedingly rapidly after bromocriptine therapy is discontinued—usually within 3 or 4 days. Some patients who derived substantial benefit from bromocriptine before developing erythromelalgia have tolerated reinstitution of therapy at 50% of their previous intake.

III. TOXICOLOGIC CONSIDERATIONS

Relevant questions about toxicity and teratology have been discussed in Chapters 2 (p. 34) and 3 (p. 86). Perhaps one toxic effect described in animals is worthy of further discussion, in view of its clinical importance. In intact female rats treated long-term with high dose bromocriptine, there was an increased incidence of endometrial and myometrial tumors. However, these effects probably reflect changes in the hormonal status in the aging female rat. Unlike women, aging female rats do not develop ovarian failure, but instead undergo either pseudopregnancy or persistent estrus owing to alterations in hypothalamic–pituitary function. During bromocriptine therapy, prolactin levels are suppressed and thus pseudopregnancy does not occur in these animals. The progesterone/estrogen ratio falls and estrogen dominance prevails. This is considered to be the explanation for uterine tumors. The observations are therefore unlikely to be relevant in the human. A study of endometrial biopsies in 88 patients who had been treated with bromocriptine for 2 to 72 months at doses varying from 1.25 to 60 mg/day did not reveal any evidence for endometrial effects of the drug. In premenopausal women, bromocriptine restores menstrual cycles and thus cystic endometrial hyperplasia or endometrial tumors are unlikely to develop. However, in women on chronic bromocriptine therapy who remain amenorrheic or are postmenopausal, it has been recommended that a full gynecologic exam, with endometrial biopsy, be performed annually so that in the unlikely event of the effects seen in rats being toxic effects of the drug, these could be diagnosed and treated before any permanent damage can occur (1).

There are neither animal nor human data to suggest that bromocriptine is teratogenic. However, until the babies born to women who took bromocriptine at the time of conception and into the early part of the pregnancy have completed their life cycles, it will not be possible to draw any final conclusions. The data up to now are encouraging *(see page 86).*

IV. CONCLUSIONS

This chapter has been devoted to considerations of adverse reaction to bromocriptine therapy. This was done to bring together the contrasting experiences of groups of physicians working in different disciplines, since the side effects differ depending on the condition for which the patient is being treated. All of the adverse effects described have led to temporary functional disturbances, which can be reversed by withdrawing therapy.

In practice, bromocriptine therapy remains extremely effective and adverse reactions are not a major problem, except in parkinsonism. It is hoped that a drug with a higher therapeutic index will be developed for treatment of parkinsonism; however, the possibility that the disease is responsible for the higher incidence of specific and severe adverse reactions may make this impossible.

REFERENCES

1. Besser, G. M., Thorner, M. O., Wass, J. A. H., Doniach, I., Canti, G., Curling, M., Grudzinskas, J. G., and Setchell, M. E. (1977): Absence of uterine neoplasia in patients on bromocriptine. *Br. Med. J.*, 2:868.
2. Besser, G. M., Wass, J. A. H., and Thorner, M. O. (1980): Bromocriptine in the medical management of acromegaly. In: *Ergot Compounds and Brain Function—Neuroendocrine and Neuropsychiatric Aspects,* edited by M. Goldstein, A. Lieberman, D. B. Calne, and M. O. Thorner. Raven Press, New York *(in press).*
3. Duvoisin, R. C., Mendoza, M. R., Yahr, M. D., and Sweet, R. D. (1979): Bromocriptine as an adjuvant to levodopa. In: *Dopaminergic Ergot Derivatives and Motor Function,* edited by K. Fuxe and D. B. Calne, pp. 329–335. Pergamon Press, Oxford.
4. Eisler, T., Hah, R. P., Kalavar, K. A. R., and Calne, D. B. (1979): Erythromelalgia-like eruption in parkinsonian patients treated with bromocriptine. *Neurology,* 29:571.
5. Klawans, H. L., Tanner, C. M., and Goetz, C. G. (1979): Psychiatric reactions to ergot derivatives. In: *Dopaminergic Ergot Derivatives and Motor Function,* edited by K. Fuxe and D. B. Calne, pp. 405–414. Pergamon Press, Oxford.
6. Sachdev, Y., Tunbridge, W. M. G., Weightman, D. R., Gomez-Pan, A., Duns, A., and Hall, R. (1975): Bromocriptine therapy in acromegaly. *Lancet,* 1:1164–1168.
7. Schran, H. F., Bhuta, S. I., Schwarz, H. J., and Thorner, M. O. (1979): The pharmacokinetics of bromocriptine. In: *Ergot Compounds and Brain Function—Neuroendocrine and Neuropsychiatric Aspects,* edited by M. Goldstein, A. Lieberman, D. B. Calne, and M. O. Thorner. Raven Press, New York *(in press).*
8. Stern, G., Lees, A., and Shaw, K. (1979): Ergot derivatives without levodopa in parkinsonism. In: *Dopaminergic Ergot Derivatives and Motor Function,* edited by K. Fuxe and D. B. Calne, pp. 337–342. Pergamon Press, Oxford.

9. Thorner, M. O., Chait, A., Aitken, M., Benker, G., Bloom, S. R., Mortimer, C. H., Sanders, P., Stuart Mason, A., and Besser, G. M. (1975): Bromocriptine treatment of acromegaly. *Br. Med. J.,* 1:299–303.
10. Valenzuela, J. E. (1976): Dopamine as a possible neurotransmitter in gastric relaxation. *Gastroenterology,* 71:1019–1022.
11. Wass, J. A. H., Thorner, M. O., and Besser, G. M. (1976): Digital vasospasm with bromocriptine. *Lancet,* 1:1135.
12. Wass, J. A. H., Thorner, M. O., Besser, G. M., Morris, D., Stuart Mason, A., Luizzi, A., and Chiodini, P. G. (1976): Gastrointestinal bleeding in patients on bromocriptine. *Lancet,* 2:851.
13. Wass, J. A. H., Thorner, M. O., Morris, D. V., Rees, L. H., Stuart Mason, A., Jones, A. E., and Besser, G. M. (1977): Long term treatment of acromegaly with bromocriptine. *Br. Med. J.,* 1:875–878.

7

Future Indications for Bromocriptine

I. INTRODUCTION

Bromocriptine has been used experimentally in the treatment of a wide variety of conditions ranging from irreversible airways obstruction (41) to anorexia nervosa (22). This chapter discusses only a few selected potential indications that have attracted wider interest or appear particularly interesting. It should be stressed that the choice of indications discussed is personal, and it is possible in the future major indications will emerge that have been omitted.

II. EFFECTS OF BROMOCRIPTINE ON PITUITARY TUMOR SIZE

The effects of bromocriptine in reducing prolactin levels to normal in patients with and without pituitary tumors were discussed in Chapter 3. The management of large pituitary tumors secreting prolactin has been unsatisfactory since surgery only rarely cures the patients, and in the few studies that have been performed, radiotherapy does not appear to restore prolactin levels to normal (page 79). However, there is now increasing evidence to show that bromocriptine can lead to a reduction in tumor size in patients with prolactin-secreting pituitary tumors. This finding is perhaps not unexpected since other ergot alkaloids, which share the property of being dopamine agonists, have been shown to inhibit growth of experimental transplantable rat pituitary tumors (34,45,46). More recently, however, Lamberts and MacLeod (28) have shown that bromocriptine is ineffective in inhibiting growth of two of these experimental tumors (MtTW15 and 7315A) and also that it does not lower prolactin levels. These observations are not altogether surprising in that these rat tumors appear to be devoid of dopamine receptors. In contrast, ergocornine, ergocristine, and ergotamine were found to be effective. These agents are presumably active through vascular mechanisms, as they are potent alpha adrenoreceptor agonists, whereas bromocriptine is an alpha adrenoreceptor antagonist. Bromocriptine has been shown to be effective in inhibiting mitosis induced by estrogen in the *in situ* rat pituitary and also in inhibiting DNA synthesis (15,33,53).

In man it has been particularly difficult to delineate and follow changes in the size of pituitary tumors without performing repeated pneumoencephalograms. The introduction both of computer tomographic (CT) scanning and of cisternography using tomography with the intrathecal water-soluble contrast medium metrizamide have facilitated the study of the effects of bromocriptine on tumor size. The promise of higher resolution CT scanners should further simplify this task.

The first suggestion that bromocriptine may have a beneficial effect in reducing tumor size came with the report of Corenblum et al. (14) of improvement of visual field defects in one patient and in pituitary function in another. Since then there have been several reports (Table 1) of reduction in tumor size by bromocriptine documented not only by improvement in visual field defects

TABLE 1. *Evidence for bromocriptine induced remission of pituitary tumors*

Reference	Age (years)	Sex	Hyperprolactinemia (P)/ Acromegaly (A)	Radiologic evaluation of tumor size	Other therapy	Bromocriptine (mg/day)	Serum prolactin (ng/ml)		Interval (months) until evidence for tumor shrinkage obtained					
							Before	On bromocriptine	Visual fields	Radiologic evidence				Improvement of anterior pituitary function
										PEG	MC	CT	SXR	
13,14	24	F	P	PEG	?	?	>3000	N	I[g]	6[a]	—	—	—	—
		F	P	SXR	?	?	↑	N	—	—	—	—	—	6
61	37	M	P	CT	Surgery	7.5	650	3	—	—	—	12	—	—
40[c]	35	F	P	SXR	—	5	49	4	—	—	—	—	I[g]	—[c]
52[d]	30	F	P	SXR	None	7.5	3760	260	—	13[b]	—	—	—	—[d]
20	30	F	P	PEG	Prednisone/thyroid	10.0	3160	20	I @ 1, N @ 8	9	—	—	—	—
	34	F	P	PEG	None	5.0	716	17	—	48	—	—	—	—
37	27	M	P	CT	Surgery and RT	20	400	150	N @ 1	—	3	3	—	3
30	56	M	P	SXR, CT	Surgery and RT	10	400	<2	—	—	11	—	—	—
62			P	SXR	RT	7.5	90	8	—	—	—	—	19	—
			P	SXR	RT	7.5	>500	<5	—	—	—	—	73	—
			P	SXR	RT	7.5	500	15	—	—	—	—	78	—
			P	SXR	—	20	>63	7	—	—	—	—	40	—
			P	SXR	—	5	60	7	—	—	—	—	27	—
			P	SXR	—	30	120	<4	I @ 2; N @ 8	—	—	—	—	—
			A,P	SXR	RT	30	78	—	—	—	—	—	31	—
			A	SXR	RT	20	9	—	—	—	—	—	12	—
			A,P	SXR	RT	30	28	—	—	—	—	—	12	—
			A	SXR	RT	15	11	—	—	—	—	—	48	—
			A	SXR	RT	10	14	—	—	—	—	—	24	—
			A,P	SXR	None	60	29	—	I @ 1	—	—	—	—	—
			A,P	SXR	None	60	63	—	I @ 3	—	—	—	—	—
			A,P	SXR, CT	None	30	90	—	—	—	—	11	—	12

38	29	M	P	SXR, CT, MC	Surgery and RT	20	379	4	—	—	3	3	—	3
	60	M	P	SXR, CT, MC	Surgery and RT	20	409	4	—	—	3	3	—	3
	50	M	P	SXR, CT, MC		20	106	6	—	—	3	3	—	3
	34	F	P	SXR, CT, MC		20	448	121	—	—	3	3	—	3
55	24	M	P	SXR, CT	None	7.5	3900	2	I < 1	—	—	0.5	—	1
	25	M	P	SXR, CT, MC	None	7.5	2350	182	—	—	1.5	—	—	—
42[e]	31	F	P	SXR	None	5–20	620	19	—	—	—	—	—	—[e]
4[f]	38	F	P	SXR	Surgery	5	3445	12	—	—	—	—	—	—[f]

[a] Ref. 13.
[b] Sphenoid sinus mass.
[c] Pituitary fossa increased in size with pregnancy and then regressed.
[d] Prolactin level only rose to 435 ng/ml after withdrawal.
[e] Operative finding of shrunken tumor.
[f] Developed CSF rhinorrhea 15 months postoperatively 5 weeks after starting bromocriptine.
[g] Interval not available.
Abbreviations: I, improved; N, normal; PEG, pneumoencephalogram; MC, metrizamide cisternography; CT, computerized tomography scanning; SXR, skull X-ray; RT, radiotherapy.

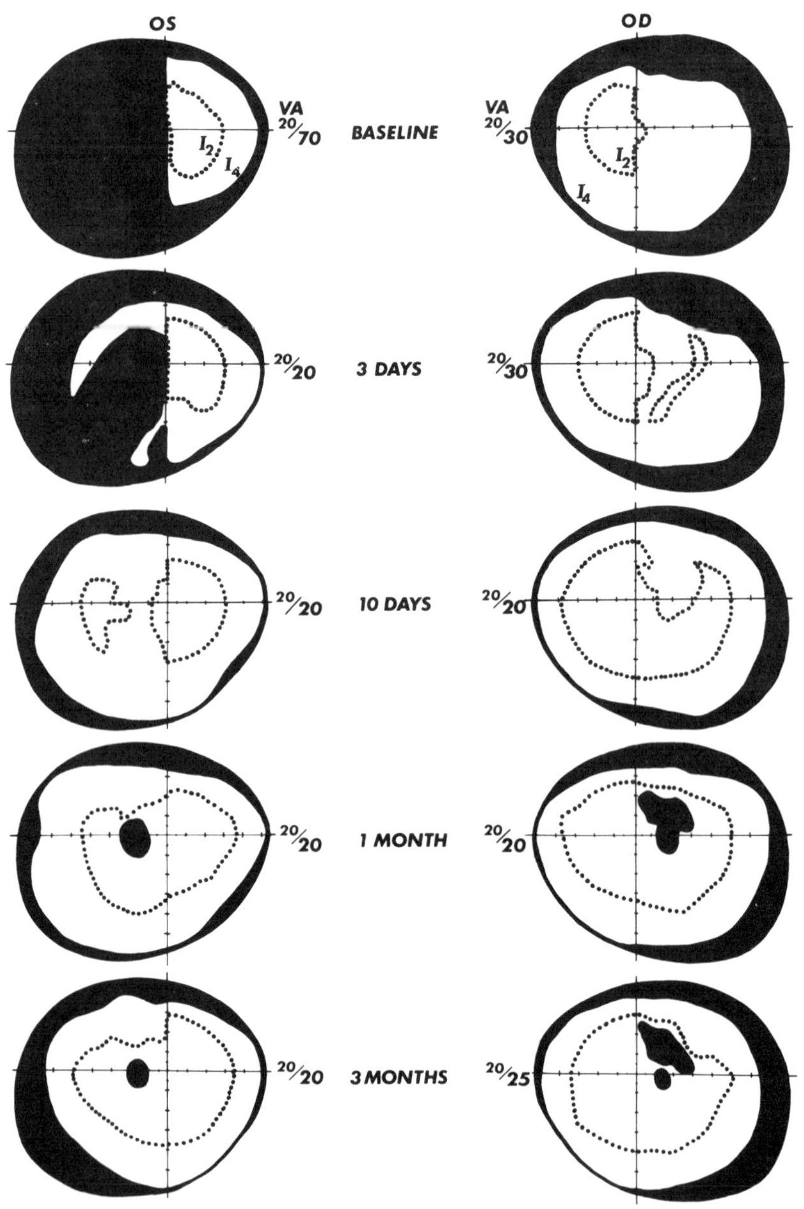
OS
OD
VA
20/70
BASELINE
VA
20/30
I_2
I_4
I_2
I_4
20/20
3 DAYS
20/30
20/20
10 DAYS
20/20
20/20
1 MONTH
20/20
20/20
3 MONTHS
20/25

(an indirect measure of tumor size), but also by radiologic means using pneumoencephalography (13,20,52), CT scans (37,38, 55,61,62), and metrizamide cisternography (37,38,55). Almost all of the patients reported to date harbored prolactin-secreting tumors, although Wass et al. (62) have reported evidence of shrinkage of growth-hormone-secreting tumors in eight patients, two of whom had been treated with bromocriptine alone. Both these patients had hyperprolactinemia prior to therapy.

The mechanism by which bromocriptine leads to tumor shrinkage is unknown. A possibility that these patients may have undergone spontaneous infarction of their tumors seems unlikely; in a number of patients there has been a return of previously deficient pituitary function (13,37,38,55,62). Furthermore, none of the patients experienced headache or other symptoms normally seen with pituitary infarction. That bromocriptine may lead to tumor regression is evidenced by the observation that following withdrawal of bromocriptine in patients with macroadenomas, prolactin levels rise once more but to lower levels than originally seen (61). Further, J. Hardy *(personal communication)* noted that at the time of surgery, tumors in bromocriptine-treated patients appear to have shrunk. This observation was also made by Nillius and colleagues (42).

We have recently had the opportunity to study two men with large pituitary tumors with extremely high prolactin levels (55).

FIG. 1. *Patient 1:* Visual acuity and diagrammatic representation of visual field plots before and during 3 months of bromocriptine therapy. The visual fields were plotted by one observer using the Goldman apparatus under identical conditions with a 0.25 mm^2 object (I) at two different light intensities, 1000 apostilb (4) and 100 apostilb (2). The *black periphery* indicates a normal visual field for comparison. Before therapy a complete temporal hemianopsia was present in the left eye, and incomplete temporal hemianopsia on the right eye, with reduced visual acuity in both. At 3 days the left visual field had improved and visual acuity was restored to 20/20. Thereafter there was progressive improvement in visual fields which were normal at 1 month except for equivocal superior bitemporal quadrantic defects to the low intensity object. (Reproduced with permission from Thorner et al., ref. 55.)

One of these patients had a large suprasellar extension with bitemporal hemianopsia. The changes in visual fields over 3 months of therapy are shown in Fig. 1. Within days of starting treatment, visual acuity and fields began to improve and were almost normal at the end of 1 month's treatment. On CT scan, the tumor had decreased in size at 2 weeks (Fig. 2). The second patient, who also had extremely high prolactin levels (2,350 ng/ml), had a large pituitary tumor with bulging of the diaphragma sellae into the chiasmatic cistern but did not demonstrate any visual field defects. After 6 weeks' treatment with bromocriptine, not only were his prolactin levels lowered to 10% of pretreatment values, but he had a partially empty fossa, as shown by metrizamide cisternography (Fig. 3). In a third patient, a large pituitary tumor was present, but the patient was ACTH and TSH deficient as well as being hyperprolactinemic. On replacement therapy with L-thyroxine and hydrocortisone together with bromocriptine therapy his tumor also became smaller, and at the end of a year he had a partially empty fossa demonstrated on metrizamide cisternography.

Thus, experience with bromocriptine indicates that at least some patients with prolactin-secreting tumors show definite evidence of tumor shrinkage with this therapy alone. Shrinkage can occur within days, and in our first patient was documented on CT scan at 2 weeks. At the present time, it is not clear how many of these tumors respond in this way, but it appears to be at least 20% (62). McGregor et al. (38) report reduction in tumor size in all five of their patients with prolactinomas. Since surgery is rarely effective in restoring prolactin levels to normal in patients with large pituitary tumors with extrasellar extension, there is a need for a controlled study to evaluate the frequency with which bromocriptine alone is able to shrink these tumors. The final role of bromocriptine, as primary treatment for large prolactinomas in the short or long term is unclear; this therapy may allow the tumor to shrink and thereby make it more amenable to permanent cure by surgery. Furthermore, this therapy can lead to recovery of anterior pituitary function; it does not appear to produce further anterior pituitary hormone deficiency, which may be seen after pituitary surgery.

III. HYPERTENSION

The effects of bromocriptine on the cardiovascular system in animals were discussed in Chapter 2. From these studies it is clear that bromocriptine does, at least transiently, lower blood pressure. In the anesthetized dog, Clark et al. (12) showed this effect to be at least partially peripherally mediated via dilitation of the renal and mesenteric vascular beds, presumably mediated by stimulation of peripheral dopamine receptors. However, dopamine mechanisms are also implicated in the modulation of the sympathetic nervous system outflow tract through both central and peripheral mechanisms (page 28). Two studies in man have shown a reduction in circulating catecholamines after bromocriptine administration (59,64). Finally, a central pathway mediating the hypotensive effect of dopamine has been proposed (23). Thus,

---

Overleaf:

FIG. 2. *Patient 1:* Coronal CT head scans (postenhancement). **Left:** Before therapy. Scan shows a large enhancing mass in the pituitary fossa extending inferiorly into sphenoid sinus and superiorly into the chiasmatic cistern and abutting onto the third ventricle (Delta 25 scanner). **Right:** Two weeks after starting bromocriptine therapy. Scan shows marked reduction in tumor size, with particular regression of the suprasellar extension. The chiasmatic cistern is now largely free of tumor apart from a finger-like process to the left of mid-line. The intrasellar high density was present in the preenhancement scan and represents calcification within the tumor (GE 8800 scanner). (Reproduced with permission from Thorner et al., ref. 55.)

FIG. 3. *Patient 2:* Tomographic sections after intrathecal metrizamide injection. **Left:** Before therapy. There is upward bulging of the diaphragma sellae into the chiasmatic cistern *(arrow)*. **Right:** Repeat study performed 6 weeks after starting bromocriptine therapy shows metrizamide within the pituitary fossa indicating cisternal herniation (partially empty fossa) due to shrinkage of the pituitary mass. (Reproduced with permission from Thorner et al., ref. 55.)

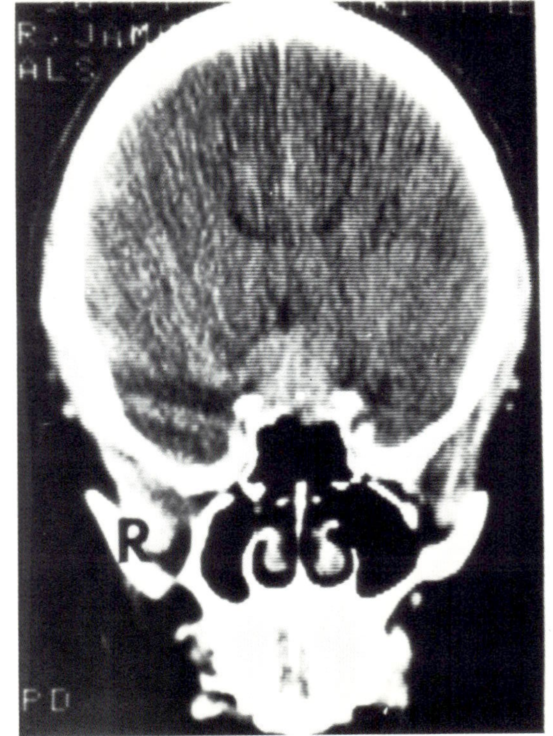

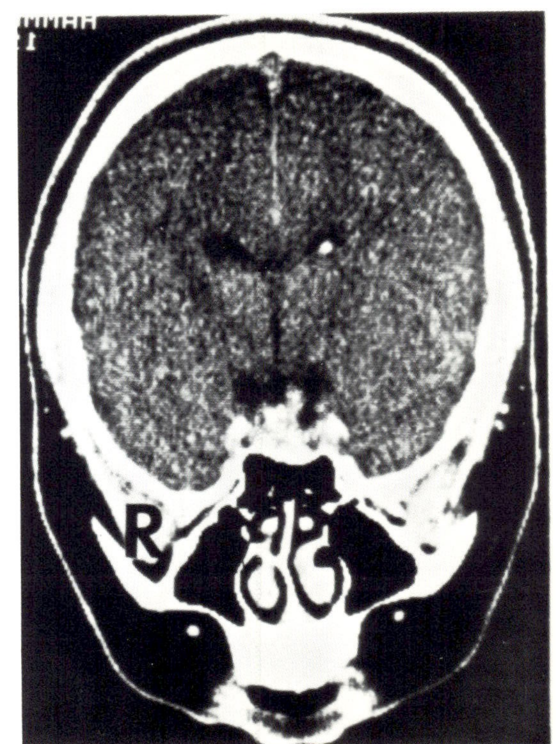

FIG. 2. Legend p. 161.

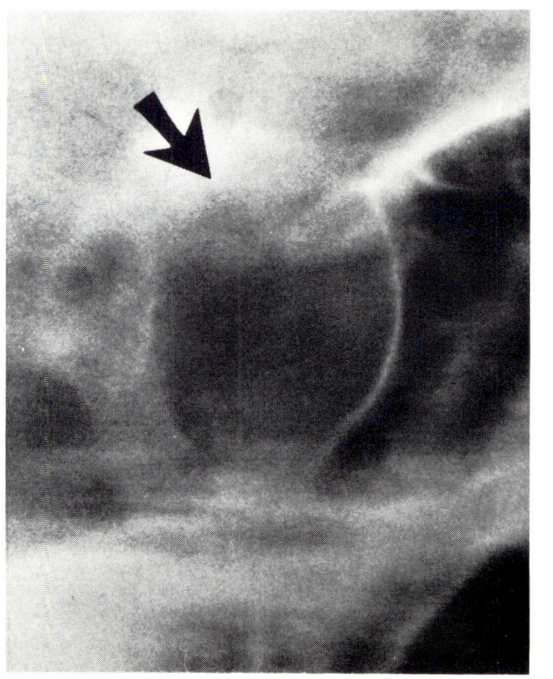

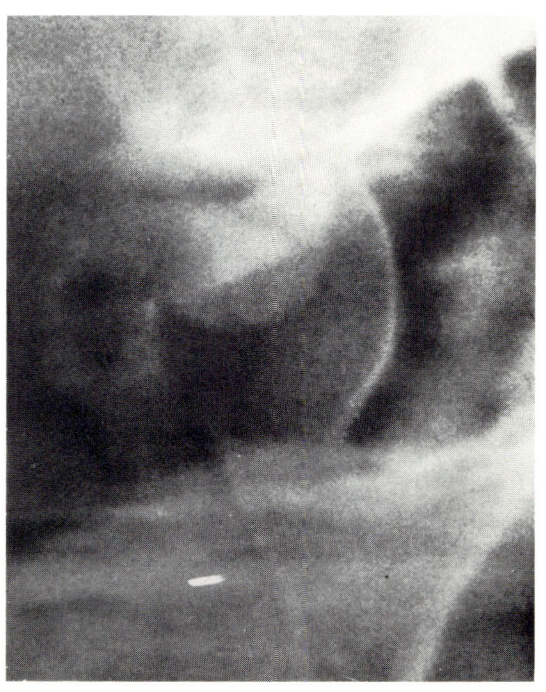

FIG. 3. Legend p. 161.

there are many theoretical reasons to suppose that the compound may be useful in the treatment of hypertension.

Only one study has reported on the use of bromocriptine in the short-term treatment of essential hypertension (54). In this study of 19 young men with essential hypertension, seven had low renin hypertension and the remaining 12 had normal or high renin hypertension. However, secondary causes for hypertension had been excluded in all subjects. Those subjects with normal or high renin hypertension had elevated serum prolactin levels and responded well to bromocriptine treatment over 4 weeks. In the low-renin group, prolactin levels were also elevated, although to a lesser degree. Furthermore, in these patients bromocriptine therapy was ineffective in lowering blood pressure. Thus the authors suggested that their patients with normal or high renin hypertension may have a defect in central catecholamine function—particularly that of dopamine—which gave rise not only to the hypertension but also to the elevated prolactin levels. Parenthetically, it is extremely unusual to find hypertension in hyperprolactinemic patients.

Dopamine mechanisms are probably also implicated in the control of aldosterone secretion. Evidence in favor of this hypothesis has come from studies with bromocriptine and metoclopramide. Edwards et al. (17) showed that the rise of aldosterone response to acute salt depletion mediated by furosemide was partially prevented by pretreatment with bromocriptine, while the rise in renin levels was unaffected. This suggested that bromocriptine might directly inhibit aldosterone secretion at the level of the adrenal cortex. This hypothesis was supported by some *in vitro* studies that showed dopamine to directly inhibit the angiotensin—induced stimulation of aldosterone secretion from dispersed bovine adrenal cells (39). Furthermore, administration of the dopamine receptor blocking agent metoclopramide resulted in marked elevation of plasma aldosterone levels in man (9,43). However, this rise in aldosterone could not be blocked by bromocriptine, and bromocriptine alone was ineffective in lowering basal plasma aldosterone levels (9,10). Thus at the present time there is evidence to support an inhibitory dopaminergic effect on aldosterone secretion. However, it is possible that the mode of inhibition may not involve the same receptors as at the pituitary, since bromocriptine is capable of antagonizing the stimulatory effect of metoclopramide on prolactin release but not on aldosterone secretion. The effects of bromocriptine have been assessed in the treatment of a small number of patients with primary hyperaldosteronism, and it appears to be ineffective (35).

The observations of elevated prolactin levels in patients with essential hypertension needs confirmation. Irrespective of the outcome of these studies, the potential use of bromocriptine as a hypotensive agent needs to be fully assessed. It may be an effective agent, and from reports of its use in hyperprolactinemia it can be confidently predicted to be well tolerated by patients without serious adverse effects.

IV. BROMOCRIPTINE TREATMENT FOR NORMOPROLACTINEMIC INFERTILITY

There have been several reports of successful treatment of infertility in women with normal prolactin levels and unexplained infertility. The study by Lenton and colleagues (31) suggested that in a carefully selected group of patients with "normal" luteal function and no apparent cause for infertility the cumulative pregnancy rate was greatly increased by bromocriptine therapy, although there was no matched control group. However, in studies in which the patients were more heterogeneous (63) or had defective luteal function (49) the results have been disappointing. In the report of Wright et al. (63), 47 women with unexplained primary infertility were randomly allocated into two groups; patients in the first group received bromocriptine, 2.5 mg b.i.d., and those in the other received a placebo for up to 6 months. Five women in the placebo group and seven in the bromocriptine group conceived—the differences in cumulative pregnancy rate between the two groups was not significant. In the report by Saunders et al. (49) fifteen patients with defective luteal phase and normal prolactin levels were treated with 15 mg bromocriptine per day. There were no differences in the progesterone levels or in the pregnancy rates in these patients. However, it should be stressed that the dose of bromocriptine may have been too high, since 7.5 mg bromocriptine per day lowers progesterone levels in normal women (51).

Thus, in contrast to the results in hyperprolactinemic subjects *(see Chapter 3),* the results of studies on bromocriptine in infertility in women with normal prolactin levels are disappointing. At the present time bromocriptine therapy in this group of patients is not recommended.

V. BROMOCRIPTINE, PREMENSTRUAL SYNDROME, AND MASTALGIA

Premenstrual syndrome is poorly defined. It is characterized by lability of mood and a sensation of body swelling which usually start 7 to 14 days before menses and are relieved at its onset. The etiology of the condition is unknown. Many different treatments have been used and none are entirely satisfactory. Horrobin et al. (24) have proposed that prolactin may be an etiologic factor, but most studies show prolactin levels to be normal in these patients (2,3). The results of therapy of premenstrual syndrome with bromocriptine are mixed. It is extremely important for such studies to be carried out in a double-blind fashion. Andersch and colleagues (2) reported encouraging results by bromocriptine, particularly on irritability. On the other hand, Andersen et al. (3) noted only mastodynia to be significantly improved. Their study emphasized the difficulties inherent in the design of such research, since many symptoms were relieved by placebo.

For the role of bromocriptine in this condition to be determined, a double-blind study on the endocrine profile is required, together with objective clinical evaluation on a daily basis in these patients, beginning prior to and continuing through placebo or bromocriptine therapy.

Mastalgia, or pain in the breast, is a common symptom of fibrocystic disease of the breast. It may occur on a cyclical basis and may be either unilateral or bilateral. Patients with mastalgia usually have normal prolactin levels. In one double-blind study (8) and three open studies (36,44,50) bromocriptine was reported to be highly effective in relieving the pain, although the mechanism through which this effect occurs is unclear. The role of prolactin in fibrocystic disease of the breast has not been determined.

VI. BROMOCRIPTINE IN IMPOTENCE

In men with hyperprolactinemia, sexual function is impaired. Testosterone levels are low, and libido and potency are reduced. Bromocriptine therapy results in a rapid return of sexual function. Several groups have noted that testosterone replacement therapy alone does not restore potency in these patients, but the addition of bromocriptine therapy to the testosterone replacement therapy is effective. Thus, bromocriptine either has a direct effect on sexual function or it acts indirectly by lowering prolactin levels.

The study of sexual impotence is difficult in man since many psychological and social factors are involved. In the majority of patients with impotence, serum prolactin levels are normal. However, the administration of many drugs leads to impotence, and many, but not all, of these compounds are effective in raising prolactin levels, e.g., phenothiazines, alpha methyldopa and reserpine. Falaschi et al. (18) administered metoclopramide (10 mg t.i.d.) to a group of five normal men in an open study and found that prolactin levels were elevated in all of them. Metoclopramide administration was associated not only with reduced sexual performance, but also with reduced volume of seminal ejaculate; the latter condition is typically seen in patients with pathological hyperprolactinemia. Following withdrawal of metoclopramide, both sexual performance and seminal volume returned to normal. Although these data suggest that metoclopramide produced its effects by increasing prolactin levels, it is also possible that it could have a direct effect on central or peripheral mechanisms involved in sexual performance.

Sexual performance involves complex neurological pathways mediated through the sympathetic and parasympathetic nervous systems peripherally as well as through pathways within the spinal cord and the brain. Bromocriptine, as discussed above, has widespread effects directly on dopamine mechanisms both within the central nervous system and at the periphery, and it may also have effects on other neuronal systems. Thus it is quite possible that it could affect sexual performance by mechanisms independent of prolactin.

Ambrosi et al. (1) studied the effects of bromocriptine on sexual function in 47 men with impotence without clinical or laboratory evidence of underlying primary organic disease responsible for their symptoms. Thirty of the patients were treated in a double-blind manner. Bromocriptine had no effects on circulating testosterone, gonadotropin, or 17-beta estradiol levels. Although 50% of the patients benefitted from bromocriptine therapy, 44% of those treated with placebo experienced a similar response. This study emphasizes the difficulty in performing such studies, since suggestion alone is extremely effective in treating impotence—psychological factors are extremely important. At the present time, bromocriptine has been shown to be effective in the treatment of sexual dysfunction in men with hyperprolactinemia, whereas it does not appear to be effective in normoprolactinemic men.

VII. CUSHING'S DISEASE

ACTH secretion is controlled by a corticotropin releasing factor (CRF), which to date has eluded isolation despite tremendous efforts by many groups. However the release of CRF is, like that of other hypothalamic regulatory hormones, under control of neurotransmitters in the hypothalamus. Over a number of years the neural control of ACTH has been extensively studied.

Ganong (19) has conducted a series of elegant studies in the dog and rat, showing that ACTH release can be inhibited by catecholamines, particularly alpha agonists. Furthermore, Van Loon et al. (60) reported that depletion of central catecholamines in the rat with reserpine or alpha methyl-para-tyrosine led to loss of circadian rhythm of corticosterone—an animal model of Cushing's disease. This could be reversed with levodopa or dihydroxyphenylserine (DOPS), suggesting either a dopaminergic or more likely an alpha adrenergic tonic inhibitory mechanism on ACTH secretion (58).

In normal man, dopamine agonists—including bromocriptine, lergotrile, and lisuride—do not produce any acute changes in cortisol, and during chronic therapy with bromocriptine, cortisol responses to insulin-induced hypoglycemia are normal (16,27, 29,56). However, methyl amphetamine, which stimulates directly or indirectly alpha and beta adrenoreceptors and probably dopamine receptors, is a potent stimulator of ACTH secretion; however, its effects are blocked by the alpha blocking agent thymoxamine, while its effects are potentiated by the beta blocking agent propranolol (6,47). Thus these data suggest that stimulation of adrenoreceptors leads to stimulation of ACTH secretion; an opposite effect to that observed in the dog or rat.

Cushing's disease, or pituitary-dependent Cushing's syndrome, is characterized by excessive ACTH secretion from the pituitary. Whether the disease is primarily pituitary or hypothalamic in origin has been widely discussed. In the majority of patients the disease is associated with a pituitary tumor which can be surgically, selectively removed with cure of the condition (11, 21,48,57). However, in a minority of patients, hyperplasia of the ACTH-secreting cells in the pituitary is found, with no distinct adenoma (11). Thus in these patients the disease may be hypothalamic in origin, leading to excessive corticotropin-releasing factor secretion. It is also possible that some adenomas may arise as a result of prolonged stimulation by CRF, i.e., hyperplasia leading to adenoma formation. Further indication that Cushing's disease may not only be caused by the development *de novo* of a pituitary tumor is that these tumors are not autonomous; they retain sensitivity to feedback by glucocorticoids, although the set point is higher (32).

There is no consensus as to the optimum therapy for Cushing's disease. We will not discuss here the advantages and disadvantages of the various modes of therapy, which include transsphenoidal selective pituitary adenoma removal, pituitary irradiation with or without bilateral adrenalectomy, and medical therapy either with enzyme blockers to inhibit cortisol synthesis or with drugs that effect neural mechanisms to modulate ACTH secretion. Krieger and colleagues (26) have pioneered the treatment of Cushing's disease with cyproheptadine, a drug thought to block 5HT receptors. Although cortisol levels were lowered, the normal circadian rhythm of ACTH was not restored by this mode of therapy.

Benker et al. (5) reported that a single 2.5 mg dose of bromocriptine could lower ACTH levels in one patient who had previously undergone bilateral adrenalectomy for Cushing's disease and in one patient with Nelson's syndrome. Similarly, Lamberts and Birkenhager (27) reported a fall in ACTH levels in six of seven patients with Cushing's disease after an acute 2.5 mg dose of bromocriptine. In other studies on Cushing's disease, Lamberts et al. (29) performed insulin tolerance tests before and 3 hr after an acute dose of bromocriptine. They found the basal ACTH levels to be lowered in all four subjects, and cortisol levels were lowered in two of three subjects in whom the levels were measured. The absent ACTH and cortisol response to hypoglycemia, normally seen in Cushing's syndrome, persisted; however, the suppressed growth hormone response was partially restored in three subjects. Four patients were treated chronically with bromocriptine (5–20 mg/day); good results with normalization of cortisol secretion rates were seen in two patients, while the cortisol secretion rate in the other two patients appeared to escape treatment. Besser et al. (7) reported three cases who showed a fall in ACTH levels while also on metyrapone therapy. One of these patients was subsequently treated with bromocriptine, 1.25 mg b.i.d., with return of the normal circadian rhythm of cortisol and a cortisol response to hypoglycemia. When she was withdrawn from therapy her Cushing's disease recurred. Similarly, Kennedy and Montgomery (25) reported encouraging results in one patient.

At the present time it appears that there are certain patients with Cushing's disease who respond well to bromocriptine. Lamberts et al. (29) suggested that depletion of central dopamine stores may be implicated in the pathophysiology of the condition. However, subsequent experience suggests that only a minority of patients with Cushing's disease respond to bromocriptine therapy. Do these patients represent a different disease process than that of the majority of patients, who do not respond? How can these patients be best identified? Currently, there does not appear to be any way in which to predict which patients will respond to bromocriptine other than performing a therapeutic trial. Cushing's disease is almost certainly heterogeneous and not due to a single etiology. As our understanding of the control of CRF and ACTH secretion in normal subjects and in patients with Cushing's disease becomes more sophisticated, it is likely that the application of bromocriptine and other drugs that modulate neural mechanisms will become more successful in the treatment of Cushing's disease.

REFERENCES

1. Ambrosi, B., Bara, R., Trawaglini, P., Weber, G., Beck Peccoz, P., Rondena, M., Elli, R., and Faglia, G. (1977): Study of the effects of bromocriptine on sexual impotence. *Clin. Endocrinol.,* 7:417–421.
2. Andersch, B., Hahn, L., Wendestan, C., Öhman, R., and Abrahamson, L. (1978): Treatment of premenstrual tension syndrome with bromocriptine. *Acta Endocrinologica (Suppl. 216),* 88:165–174.
3. Andersen, A. N., Larsen, J. F., Steenstrup, O. R., Svendstrup, B., and Nielsen, J. (1977): Effect of bromocriptine on the premenstrual syndrome. *Br. J. Obstet. Gynaecol.,* 84:370–374.
4. Aronoff, S. L., Daughaday, W. H., and Laws, E. R. (1979): Bromocriptine treatment of prolactinomas. *N. Engl. J. Med.,* 300:1391.
5. Benker, G., Hackenberg, K., Hamburger, B., and Reinwein, D. (1976): Effects of growth hormone release-inhibiting hormone and bromocriptine

(CB-154) in states of abnormal pituitary-adrenal function. *Clin. Endocrinol.,* 5:187–190.

6. Besser, G. M., Butler, P. W. P., Landon, J., and Rees, L. H. (1969): Influence of amphetamines on plasma corticosteroid and growth hormone levels in man. *Br. Med. J.,* 4:528–530.
7. Besser, G. M., Jeffcoate, W. J., and Tomlin, S. (1976): The use of metyrapone and bromocriptine in the control of Cushing's syndrome. *Abstracts of the Vth International Congress of Endocrinology,* Hamburg, July 18–24, Abstract 494.
8. Blichert-Toft, M., Andersen, A. N., Henriksen, O. B., and Mygind, T. (1979): Treatment of mastalgia with bromocriptine: A double blind cross-over study. *Brit. Med. J.,* 1:237.
9. Carey, R. M., Thorner, M. O., and Ortt, E. M. (1979): Effects of metoclopramide and bromocriptine on the renin-angiotensin-aldosterone system in man: Dopaminergic control of aldosterone. *J. Clin. Invest.,* 63:727–735.
10. Carey, R. M., Thorner, M. O., and Ortt, B. Dopaminergic inhibition of metoclopramide induced aldosterone secretion in man. *(In preparation).*
11. Carmalt, M. H. B., Dalton, G. A., Fletcher, R. F., and Thomas Smith, W. (1977): The treatment of Cushing's disease by trans-sphenoidal hypophysectomy. *Q. J. Med,* 46:119–134.
12. Clarke, B. J., Scholtysik, G., and Flückiger, E. (1978): Cardiovascular actions of bromocriptine. *Acta Endocrinologica (Suppl. 216),* 88:75–81.
13. Corenblum, B. (1978): Bromocriptine in pituitary tumors. *Lancet,* 2:786.
14. Corenblum, B., Webster, B. R., Mortimer, C. B., and Ezrin, C. (1975): Possible anti-tumor effect of 2-bromo-ergocryptine (CB-154, Sandoz) in two patients with large prolactin secreting pituitary adenomas. *Clin. Res.,* 23:614A.
15. Davies, C., Jacobi, J., Lloyd, H. M., and Meares, J. D. (1974): DNA synthesis and secretion of prolactin and growth hormone by the pituitary gland of the male rat: Effects of diethyl stilboestrol and 2-brom-α-ergokryptine methane-sulphanate. *J. Endocrinol.,* 61:411–417.
16. Delitala, G., Wass, J. A. H., Stubbs, W. A., Jones, A., Williams, S., and Besser, G. M. (1979): The effects of lisuride hydrogen maleate, an ergot derivative on anterior pituitary hormone secretion in man. *Clin. Endocrinol.,* 11:1–9.
17. Edwards, C. R. W., Thorner, M. O., Miall, P. A., Al-Dujaili, E. A. S., Hanker, J. P., and Besser, G. M. (1975): Inhibition of plasma aldosterone response to frusemide by bromocriptine. *Lancet,* 2:903–905.
18. Falaschi, P., Frajese, G., Sciarra, F., Rocco, A., and Conti, C. (1978): Influence of hyperprolactinemia due to metoclopramide on gonadal function in men. *Clin. Endocrinol.,* 8:427–433.
19. Ganong, W. F. (1975): Brain amines and the control of ACTH and growth hormone secretion. In: *Hypothalamic Hormones: Chemistry, Physiology, Pharmacology and Clinic Usage,* edited by M. Motta, T. G. Crosignani, and L. Martini, pp. 237–248. Academic Press, New York.
20. George, S. R., Burrow, G. N., Zinman, B., and Ezrin, C. (1979): Regression

of pituitary tumors, a possible effect of bromergocryptine. *Am. J. Med.*, 66:697–702.

21. Hardy, J. (1973): Transsphenoidal surgery of hypersecreting pituitary tumors. In: *Diagnosis and Treatment of Pituitary Tumors,* edited by P. O. Kohler and G. T. Ross, pp. 179–194. American Elsevier, New York.
22. Harrower, A. D., Yat, P. L., Nairn, I. M., Walton, H. J., Strong, J. A., and Craig, A. (1977): Growth hormone, insulin, and prolactin secretion in anorexia nervosa and obesity during bromocriptine treatment. *Br. Med. J.*, 2:156–159.
23. Heise, A. (1976): Hypotensive action of central α-adrenergic and dopaminergic receptors stimulation. In: *New Antihypertensive Drugs,* edited by E. A. Scriabine and C. S. Sweet, pp. 135–145. Spectrum Publications Inc, New York.
24. Horrobin, D. F., Manku, M. S., Nassar, B., and Evered, D. (1973): Prolactin and fluid and electrolyte balance. In: *Human Prolactin,* edited by J. L. Pasteels and C. Robyn, pp. 152–155. American Elsevier, New York.
25. Kennedy, A. L., and Montgomery, D. A. D. (1977): Bromocriptine for Cushing's disease. *Br. Med. J.*, 1:1084–1085.
26. Krieger, D. T., Amorosa, L., and Linick, F. (1975): Cyproheptadine-induced remission of Cushing's disease. *N. Engl. J. Med.*, 293:893–896.
27. Lamberts, S. W. J. and Birkenhager, J. C. (1976): Effect of bromocriptine in pituitary-dependent Cushing's syndrome. *J. Endocrinol.*, 70:315–316.
28. Lamberts, S. W. J., and MacLeod, R. M. (1979): The inability of bromocriptine to inhibit prolactin secretion by transplantable rat pituitary tumors. *Endocrinology,* 104:65–71.
29. Lamberts, S. W. J., Timmermans, H. A. T., De Jong, F. H., and Birkenhager, J. C. (1977): The role of dopaminergic depletion in the pathogenesis of Cushing's disease and the possible consequences for medical therapy. *Clin. Endocrinol.*, 7:185–193.
30. Landolt, A. M., Wuthrich, R., and Fellmann, H. (1979): Regression of pituitary prolactinoma after treatment. *Lancet,* 1:1082–1083.
31. Lenton, E. A., Sobowale, O. S., and Cooke, I. D. (1977): Prolactin concentrations in ovulatory but infertile women: Treatment with bromocriptine. *Br. Med. J.*, 2:1179–1181.
32. Liddle, G. W. (1960): Tests of pituitary-adrenal suppressibility in the diagnosis of Cushing's syndrome. *J. Clin. Endocrinol. Metab.*, 20:1539–1560.
33. Lloyd, H. M., Meares, J. D., and Jacobi, J. (1975): Effects of estrogen and bromocriptine on *in vivo* secretion and mitosis in prolactin cells. *Nature,* 255:497–498.
34. MacLeod, R. M., and Lehmeyer, J. E. (1973): Suppression of pituitary tumor growth and function by ergot alkaloids. *Cancer Res.*, 33:849–855.
35. Marek, J., and Horky, K. (1976): Bromocriptine and plasma aldosterone. *Lancet,* 2:1409.
36. Martin-Comin, J., Pujol-Amat, P., Cararach, V., Davi, E., and Robyn, C. (1976): Treatment of fibrocystic diasease of the breast (CB-154) with a prolactin inhibitor: 2-Br-alpha-ergocryptine. *Obstet. Gynecol.*, 48:703–706.

37. McGregor, A. M., Scanlon, M. F., Hall, K., Cook, D. B., and Hall, R. (1979): Reduction in size of a pituitary tumor by bromocriptine therapy. *N. Engl. J. Med.,* 300:291–293.
38. McGregor, A. M., Scanlon, M. F., Hall, R., and Hall, K. (1979): Effects of bromocriptine on pituitary tumour size. *Br. Med. J.,* 2:700–703.
39. McKenna, T. J., Island, D. P., and Nicholson, W. F. (1979): Dopamine inhibits angiotensin-stimulated aldosterone biosynthesis in bovine adrenal cells. *J. Clin. Invest.,* 64:287–291.
40. Mühlenstedt, D., Osmers, F. and Schneider, H. P. G. (1978): Regression eines Hypophysenadenoms unter Bromocriptin. *Arch. Gynecol.,* 226:341–346.
41. Newman-Taylor, A. J., Soutar, C., Sheerson, J., and Turner Warwick, M. (1976): Paper read at the Thoracic Society Meeting, Liverpool, July 15–16.
42. Nillius, S. J., Bergh, T., Lundbergh, P. O., Stahle, J., and Wide, L. (1978): Regression of a prolactin-secreting pituitary tumor during long-term treatment with bromocriptine. *Fertil. Steril.,* 30:710–712.
43. Norbiato, G., Bevilacqua, M., Raggi, U., Micossi, P., and Moroni, C. (1977): Metoclopramide increases plasma aldosterone in man. *J. Clin. Endocrinol. Metab.,* 45:1313–1316.
44. Palmer, B. V., and Monteiro, J. C. M. P. (1977): Bromocriptine for severe mastalgia. *Br. Med. J.,* 1:1083.
45. Quadri, S. K., and Meites, J. (1972): Ergot induced inhibition of pituitary tumor growth in rats. *Science,* 176:417–418.
46. Quadri, S. K., and Meites, J. (1973): Effects of ergocornine and CG 603 on blood prolactin and growth hormone in rats bearing a pituitary tumor. *Proc. Soc. Exp. Biol. Med.,* 142:837–841.
47. Rees, L. H., Butler, P. W. P., Gosling, C., and Besser, G. M. (1970): Adrenergic blockade and the corticosteroid and growth hormone responses to methylamphetamine. *Nature,* 228:565–566.
48. Salassa, R. M., Laws, E. R., Carpenter, P. C., and Northcutt, R. C. (1978): Transsphenoidal removal of pituitary microadenoma in Cushing's disease. *Mayo Clin. Proc.,* 53:24–28.
49. Saunders, D. B., Hunter, J. C., Haase, H. R. and Wilson, G. R. (1979): Treatment of luteal phase inadequacy with bromocriptine. *Obstet. Gynecol.,* 53:287–289.
50. Schultz, K-D., Del Pozo, E., Lose, K. H., Künzig, H. J., and Geiger, W., (1975): Successful treatment of mastodynia with the prolactin inhibitor bromocryptine (CB-154). *Archiv. Gynäkologie,* 220:83–87.
51. Schultz, K.-D., Geiger, W., Del Pozo, E., and Künzig, H. J. (1978): Pattern of sexual steroids, prolactin and gonadotropin hormones during prolactin inhibition in normally cycling women. *Am. J. Obstet. Gynecol.* 132:561–566.
52. Sobrinho, L. G., Nunes, M. C. P., Santos, M. A., and Manricio, J. C. (1978): Radiological evidence for regression of prolactinoma after treatment with bromocriptine. *Lancet,* 2:257–258.

53. Stepien, H., Wolanink, A., and Pawlikowski, M. (1978): Effects of pimozide and bromocriptine on anterior pituitary cell proliferation. *J. Neural Transmiss.*, 42:239–244.
54. Stumpe, L. O., Kohoch, R., Higuchi, M., Krück, F., and Vetter, H. (1977): Hyperprolactinemia and antihypertensive effect of bromocriptine in essential hypertension. *Lancet*, 2:211–214.
55. Thorner, M. O., Martin, W. H., Rogol, A. D., Morris, J. L., Perryman, R. L., Conway, B. P., Howards, S. S., Wolfman, M. G., and MacLeod, R. M. Rapid regression of pituitary prolactinomas during bromocriptine treatment. *(Submitted for publication.)*
56. Thorner, M. O., Ryan, S. M., Wass, J. A. H., Jones, A., Bouloux, P., Williams, S., and Besser, G. M. (1978): Effect of the dopamine agonist lergotrile mesylate on the circulating anterior pituitary hormones in man. *J. Clin. Endocrinol. Metab.*, 47:372–378.
57. Tyrrell, J. B., Brooks, R. M., Fitzgerald, P. A., Cofoid, P. B., Forsham, P. H., and Wilson, C. B. (1978): Cushing's disease: Selective trans-sphenoidal resection of pituitary microadenomas. *N. Engl. J. Med.*, 298:753–758.
58. Van Loon, G. R. (1973): Brain catecholamines and ACTH secretion. In: *Frontiers in Neuroendocrinology*, edited by W. F. Ganong and L. Martini, pp. 209–242. Oxford University Press, New York.
59. Van Loon, G. R. (1978): A defect in catecholamine neurons in patients with prolactin secreting adenomas. *Lancet*, 2:868–871.
60. Van Loon, G. R., Nicholson, W., and Brown, R. (1971): Drug induced hypersecretion of ACTH in rats and treatment with L-dopa. *Program of the 53rd Meeting of the Endocrine Society*, Abstract 129.
61. Von Werder, K., Brendel, C., Eversmann, T., Fahlbusch, R., Müller, O. A., and Rjosk, H. K. (1979): Medical therapy of hyperprolactinemia and Cushing's disease associated with pituitary adenomas. In: *Pituitary Microadenomas*, edited by G. Faglia, M. A. Giovanelli, and R. M. MacLeod. Academic Press, London *(in press)*.
62. Wass, J. A. H., Thorner, M. O., Charlesworth, M., Moult, P. J. A., Dacie, J. E., Jones, A. E., and Besser, G. M. (1979): Reduction of pituitary tumour size in patients with prolactinomas and acromegaly treated with bromocriptine with or without radiotherapy. *Lancet*, 2:66–69.
63. Wright, C. S., Steele, S. J., and Jacobs, H. S. (1979): Value of bromocriptine in unexplained primary infertility: A double blind controlled study. *Br. Med. J.*, 1:1037–1039.
64. Ziegler, M. G., Lake, C. R., Williams, A. C., Techenne, P. F., Shoulson, I., and Steinsland, O. (1979): Bromocriptine inhibits norepinephrine release *Clin. Pharmacol. Ther.*, 25:137–142.

Subject Index